Aids to Postgraduate Surgery

Roger M Watkins
MChir, FRCS

Consultant Surgeon
Derriford Hospital, Plymouth
(formerly Senior Surgical Registrar, Westminster Hospital and
The Royal Marsden Hospital, London)

J Meirion Thomas
MS, MRCP, FRCS

Consultant Surgeon
Westminster Hospital, London

Orthopaedic contribution by:
Peter A N Hutton
FRCS

Consultant Orthopaedic Surgeon
St Stephen's Hospital and Queen Mary's Hospital, Roehampton,
London

THIRD EDITION

CHURCHILL LIVINGSTONE
EDINBURGH LONDON MELBOURNE AND NEW YORK 1989

CHURCHILL LIVINGSTONE
Medical Division of Longman Group UK Limited

Distributed in the United States of America by Churchill Livingstone Inc.;
1560 Broadway, New York, N.Y. 10036, and by associated companies,
branches and representatives throughout the world.

First Edition 1976
Second Edition 1982
Third Edition 1989

ISBN 0-443-03807-4

British Library Cataloguing in Publication Data
Watkins, Roger M.
    Aids to postgraduate surgery. – 3rd ed.
    1. Medicine. Surgery
    I. Title. II. Hutton, Peter A.N. III. Thomas, J. Meirion (Joseph Meirion)
    IV. Thomas, J. Meirion (Joseph Meirion). Aids to postgraduate surgery
    617

Library of Congress Cataloging in Publication Data
Watkins, Roger M.
    Aids to postgraduate surgery. – 3rd edn./Roger M. Watkins, Peter A. N.
    Hutton, J. Meirion Thomas.
    p. cm.
    Rev. ed. of: Aids to postgraduate surgery/J. Meirion Thomas, John S.
    Belstead. 2nd ed. 1982.
    Includes bibliographies and index.
    ISBN 0-443-03807-4
    1. Surgery – Outlines, syllabi, etc. I. Hutton, Peter A. N. II. Thomas, J.
    Meirion (Joseph Meirion) III. Thomas, J. Meirion (Joseph Meirion) Aids to
    postgraduate surgery. IV. Title.
    [DNLM: 1. Surgery – outlines. WO 18 W335a]
    RD37.3.W37 1989
    617 – dc19
    DNLM/DLC
    for Library of Congress   88-30232

Produced by Longman Singapore Publishers (Pte) Ltd.
Printed in Singapore

Aids to Postgraduate Surgery

Preface

It is an essential prerequisite of a surgeon that, apart from basic practical surgical ability, he or she must be able to appraise the relative merits of various forms of management. The surgical examinations of the Royal Colleges are particularly biased in this direction. The surgical trainee will gain a large amount of knowledge from standard textbooks. This knowledge is then complemented by clinical experience, discussion, case presentations, clinical audit meetings, postgraduate lectures and extensive perusal of the many journals now available.

This text attempts to review the most recent opinions and developments in surgery and guides the reader to some key references where more detailed considerations might be sought. The search for references is often time-consuming and tedious. The references selected have been drawn wherever possible from the more commonly available journals. Many are review articles rather than papers reporting original work. In addition, several chapters in recent books have been quoted and we hope that all the references will be of benefit to the reader. References are not listed in any order of merit but in alphabetical order by the first authors' surnames.

In this third edition, the selection of topics is again based mainly upon areas of current controversy in surgery. The number of topics has been greatly increased reflecting many of the recent advances in surgery since the second edition was published in 1982. The chapters on percutaneous nephrolithotomy, extracorporeal shock wave lithotripsy, transluminal angioplasty and monoclonal antibodies are just a few examples of new topics included in this edition. However, all chapters have been extensively revised to include recent changes in surgical practice.

This book is intended mainly for the postgraduate student preparing for the FRCS examination but it will also be of interest and help to senior medical students.

1989
RMW
JMT

Acknowledgements

We wish to thank the many colleagues who have helped in the preparation of this book by their advice and criticism. In particular we wish to thank Professor Gerald Westbury, Professor Richard Wood, Mr Michael Pittam, Mr Mark Fordham and Mr Neil McLean for their advice in the preparation of those chapters covering thyroid tumours, organ transplantation and immunosuppression, vascular surgery, urology and burns and reconstructive surgery.

Gratitude must also be expressed to our wives and families for their tolerance in the months during which the book was written.

Contents

Upper gastro-intestinal surgery

OESOPHAGO-GASTRO-DUODENOSOCOPY

Technique
1. An invaluable technique used in the diagnosis and treatment of various upper gastro-intestinal conditions
2. Carried out using a forward viewing flexible endoscope which allows visualisation of the oesophagus, stomach and first two parts of the duodenum
3. Performed under sedation with intra-venous benzodiazepines having sprayed the oropharynx with local anaesthetic

Indications for diagnostic endoscopy
1. As an adjunct or alternative to barium meal examination in the investigation of dysphagia, reflux oesophagitis, dyspepsia, weight loss and anaemia
2. As a preliminary to surgery to the oesophagus, stomach or duodenum
3. Investigation of acute upper gastro-intestinal haemorrhage
   a. Endoscopy is the most accurate diagnostic method
   b. Barium meal examination rarely shows stomal ulcers or superficial gastric erosions and does not identify which lesion is the source of haemorrhage
4. Biopsy and brush cytology of oesophageal strictures
5. Biopsy of gastric ulcers and tumours
6. Endoscopic assessment of patients with post-gastrectomy and post-vagotomy symptoms is vital
   a. Stomal ulcers
   b. Bile gastritis
   c. Carcinoma of the gastric remnant

Indications for therapeutic endoscopy
1. Dilatation of benign oesophageal strictures
   a. A spring-tipped guide wire is passed under direct vision down the endoscope and through the stricture.
   b. Following removal of the endoscope graduated Eder-Puestow dilators are threaded over the guide wire and pushed gently through the stricture

2. Balloon dilatation of achalasia of the cardia (cardiospasm)
3. Palliative intubation of malignant oesophageal and cardial strictures
   a. The morbidity and mortality of endoscopic intubation is much less than that of surgical placement of endoprostheses
   b. The advantages are especially apparent in elderly and severely malnourished patients
      Refer to Pages 10–11
4. Injection sclerotherapy of oesophageal varices
   Refer to Page 60
5. Extraction of foreign bodies
6. Diathermy snare polypectomy
7. Laser photocoagulation and diathermy coagulation of bleeding peptic ulcers
8. Laser destruction of obstructing oesophageal and gastric neoplasms
   a. A limited number of patients unsuitable for other forms of treatment may achieve benefit from laser therapy
   b. Several have undergone palliative laser recanalisation of obstructing tumours of the oesophagus or stomach
9. Insertion of naso-enteral feeding tubes

Complications
1. Sore throat due to superficial pharyngeal trauma
2. Hypersensitivity to sedative drugs especially benzodiazepines and opiates may lead to various cardio-respiratory problems
3. Thrombophlebitis at site of intra-venous injection of benzodiazepines may be reduced by using diazepam in lipid emulsion (Diazemuls)
4. Aspiration pneumonia can be avoided by ensuring the stomach is empty prior to the endoscopic examination
5. Oesophageal perforation

FURTHER READING

Cotton P B, Bowden T A 1986 Gastrointestinal endoscopy and the surgeon. In: Russell R C G (ed) Recent Advances in Surgery 12. Churchill Livingstone, Edinburgh pp 71–88
Swain C P, Bown S G, Edwards D A W, Kirkham J S, Salmon P R, Clark C G 1984 Laser recanalisation of obstructing foregut cancer. Br J Surg 71: 112–115
McFarland J 1983 Endoscopic views of the foregut. Hosp Update 9: 1171–1182
Misiewicz J J, Bartram C I, Cotton P B, Mee A S, Price A B, Thompson R P H 1986 Diseases of the oesophagus, stomach and duodenum: a guide to diagnosis. Gower Medical Publishing, London
Vicary F R 1982 Gastroenterology: New Techniques. Hosp Update 8: 1117–1123

HIATUS HERNIA AND GASTRO-OESOPHAGEAL REFLUX

Classification of hiatus hernia
1. Sliding hernia
   a. The oesophago-gastric junction lies above the diaphragm having passed through the oesophageal hiatus
   b. As a result of incompetence of the oesophago-gastric junction reflux of gastric contents into the oesophagus occurs and the complications of reflux oesophagitis, oesophageal stricture and shortening are likely to follow
2. Para-oesophageal (rolling) hernia
   a. The apex of the hernia is formed by the gastric fundus which herniates alongside the lower oesophagus
   b. The oesophago-gastric junction remains within the abdomen and gastro-oesophageal reflux does not occur

Factors in maintaining competence of the oesophago-gastric junction
1. Intrinsic functional lower oesophageal sphincter
2. Length of intra-abdominal oesophagus which is compressed by the positive (intra-abdominal) pressure of the abdomen, its lumen being at a negative (intra-thoracic) pressure
3. Pinch-cock effect of right crus of the diaphragm on the intra-abdominal oesophagus
4. Oblique insertion of oesophagus into the stomach creating the angle of His.

Investigations
1. Barium swallow and meal
2. Endoscopy, biopsy and brush cytology
3. Oesophageal pH measurements
   a. Ambulatory (24 hour) pH monitoring
   b. Standard acid reflux test
   c. Acid clearance test
4. Oesophageal manometry
5. Radio-isotope scintigraphy

Conservative treatment of gastro-oesophageal reflux and reflux oesophagitis
The majority of symptomatic patients can be treated successfully using the following therapeutic measures.
1. Weight loss
2. Stop smoking
3. Maintenance of correct posture which avoids stooping and lying flat especially after meals
4. Raise head of bed and sleep propped upright with extra pillows
5. Avoid physical straining
6. Take small frequent meals and avoid late evening meals and drinks

7. Avoid constricting clothes
8. Antacids, e.g. magnesium trisilicate, aluminium hydroxide will neutralise excessive gastric acid but may exacerbate the symptoms in those patients with bile reflux
9. H_2-receptor antagonists, e.g. cimetidine (Tagamet), ranitidine (Zantac), by reducing gastric acid production will also help many patients but they will have no effect in cases of oesophagitis due to bile reflux
10. Cholinergic drugs, e.g. bethanechol (Myotonine) increase lower oesophageal pressure
11. Metoclopramide (Maxolon, Primperan) increases lower oesophageal sphincter tone and accelerates gastric emptying
12. Local anaesthetics combined with antacids, e.g. Mucaine, provide rapid symptomatic relief from reflux oesophagitis
13. Silicones e.g. Asilone, Polycrol reduce surface tension and therefore promote the clearance of refluxed gastric contents from the oesophagus
14. Alginates, e.g. Gastrocote, Gaviscon, Algicon, are designed to float on top of the gastric contents so that if reflux does occur the alginate 'raft' rather than gastric acid comes into contact with oesophageal mucosa

Indications for surgical treatment
1. Failure to control symptoms with conservative measures
2. Intractable oesophagitis complicated by haemorrhage or chronic anaemia
3. Oesophageal stricture which cannot be managed satisfactorily by repeated endoscopic dilation
   Refer to page 1
4. Respiratory complications secondary to tracheo-bronchial aspiration of oesophageal contents
5. Huge hiatus hernia causing post-prandial cardio-respiratory distress

Aims of surgical treatment
The surgical procedures designed to treat sliding hiatus hernias with gastro-oesophageal reflux aim to achieve one or more of the following objectives:
1. Narrow oesophageal hiatus to prevent recurrent herniation
2. Reconstitute the oesophago-gastric angle
3. Anchor the oesophago-gastric junction in a subdiaphragmatic position thereby producing a length of intra-abdominal oesophagus
4. Provide adequate gastric drainage in those cases with evidence of gastric outflow obstruction
5. Reduce any gastric acid hypersecretion by an appropriate form of vagotomy

Specific surgical procedures
1. Nissen fundoplication
   a. Performed through an upper midline abdominal incision
   b. Hiatus hernia is fully reduced
   c. The upper part of the greater curvature of the stomach is mobilised by careful division of the short gastric vessels thus avoiding damage to the spleen
   d. A large bore (50FG) gastric tube is passed by the anaesthetist into the oesophagus so that its tip lies in the body of the stomach: this prevents too tight a closure of the oesophageal hiatus
   e. Oesophageal hiatus is repaired by approximation of the two limbs of the right diaphragmatic crus
   f. The mobilised fundus is passed behind the oesophagus and through a window in the gastro-hepatic ligament above the hepatic branch of the anterior vagus
   g. Fundus is plicated anterior to the distal 3–4 cm of oesophagus starting at the oesophago-gastric junction to produce an 'unspillable inkwell'
2. Belsey Mark IV procedure
   a. An anterior fundoplication performed as trans-thoracic procedure through the left sixth intercostal space
   b. Following mobilisation of the oesophagus the fundus and upper part of the body of the stomach are folded and fixed firmly to the anterior two-thirds of the oesophagus along its most distal 3–5 cm
   c. Following reduction of the plicated oesophagus into the abdominal cavity the hiatus is narrowed with several mattress sutures
3. Collis gastroplasty
   a. Used when a shortened oesophagus prevents full reduction of the hiatus hernia
   b. Performed via a left thoraco-abdominal incision
   c. A tube formed from the proximal part of the lesser curvature lengthens the distal oesophagus and creates a new 'oesophago-gastric junction'
   d. The procedure may be performed easily using a stapling device
   e. The new fundic pouch can be used to perform a modified fundoplication
   f. The 'uncut Collis' operation produces equivalent results
4. Boerema gastropexy (anterior gastropexy)
   a. Anterior surface of the stomach close to the lesser curve is fixed to the linea alba
   b. A rapid, simple and safe procedure performed via the abdominal route
   c. Repair of the hiatus hernia is not always required

5. Hill procedure (median arcuate posterior gastropexy)
6. Angelchick anti-reflux prosthesis
   a. The lower oesophagus is fully mobilised to allow insertion of the prosthesis
   b. The C-shaped silicone gel-filled device is placed around the gastro-oesophageal junction and secured by two tapes
   c. Improvement in symptoms is due to improved function of the lower oesophageal sphincter by posterior padding of the gastro-oesophageal junction
   d. Recurrent symptoms are usually due to technical complications
   e. Displacement of the prosthesis within the peritoneal cavity follows disruption of the securing tapes
   f. Migration of the prosthesis into the mediastinum causes angulation of the oesophagus and dysphagia
7. Oesophageal resection
   a. Indications include the presence of malignancy or the development of a benign oesophageal stricture which can neither be endoscopically dilated nor mobilised at surgery
   b. Resection of the middle and lower thirds of the oesophagus is followed by oesophago-gastrostomy or replacement by a Roux-en-Y jejunal loop or transposed colon

Advantages of trans-abdominal over trans-thoracic repair of hiatus hernias
1. Post-operative morbidity and mortality of laparotomy is less than thoracotomy especially in obese middle aged and elderly patients.
2. Other intra-abdominal viscera can be readily examined.
3. Surgery for any associated conditions such as cholelithiasis and duodenal ulceration can be performed through the same incision

FURTHER READING

Celestin L R 1986 The surgical treatment of hiatus hernia and gastro-oesophageal reflux. In: Russell R C G (ed) Recent Advances in Surgery — 12. Churchill Livingstone, Edinburgh pp 89–104
Evans D F 1987 Twenty-four hour ambulatory pH monitoring: an update. Br J Surg 74: 157–161
DeMeester T R 1986 Surgical management of gastroesophageal reflux. Curr Con Gastroenterol 4: 19–24
Ott D J, McCallum R W, Skinner D B 1986 Management of gastroesophageal reflux. Curr Con Gastroenterol 4: 3–16
Thomas J M 1983 Management of hiatus hernia and reflux oesophagitis. Hosp Update 9: 1129–1142
Weaver R M, Temple J G 1985 The Angelchik prosthesis for gastro-oesophageal reflux: symptomatic and objective assessment. Ann R Coll Surg 67: 299–302

OESOPHAGEAL CARCINOMA

Pathology
1. The majority of oesophageal carcinomas are squamous in nature
2. Less than 5% are adenocarcinomas; these occur in the lower third of the oesophagus and are difficult to differentiate from gastric carcinomas arising from the cardia and directly invading the oesophagus

Prognosis
1. The overall prognosis of oesophageal carcinoma is very poor
2. Fewer than 30% of patients will survive 1 year and the 5-year survival is only 5–10%
3. Several factors account for these low survival figures.
   a. Many patients have incurable disease at the time of presentation
   b. Only a minority of patients have disease localised to the oesophagus; these are the only patients in whom curative surgery is feasible
   c. Oesophageal carcinoma often occurs in old patients with chronic cardio-respiratory disease who rapidly become malnourished and debilitated as their dysphagia worsens; an appreciable delay between the onset of dysphagia and presentation often occurs
   d. En bloc radical resection is only possible for those tumours arising in the lower third of the oesophagus.
   e. Oesophagectomy continues to be associated with a high operative mortality, in many series up to 20%
   f. Radiotherapy is often limited by the poor tolerance of the surrounding vital structures, especially the spinal cord and myocardium, to ionising radiation

Pre-malignant lesions of the oesophagus
1. Plummer–Vinson syndrome (chronic iron deficiency in women with oesophageal webs predisposing to post-cricoid carcinoma)
2. Achalasia of the cardia
3. Corrosive oesophagitis
4. Gastro-oesophageal reflux
   a. Peptic stricture
   b. Barrett's oesophagus

Subdivisions of the oesophagus
The oesophagus commences at the lower border of the hypopharynx approximately 10 cm from the incisor teeth. It is approximately 30 cm long ending at the cardia which is normally situated 40 cm from the incisor teeth. Surgically the oesophagus can be divided into three equal segments. Each third of the

oesophagus is therefore approximately 10 cm long. The relative frequencies with which tumours arise in each segment are given.
1. Upper third: crico-pharyngeus to aortic arch (20%)
   true cervical oesophagus
   supra-aortic oesophagus
2. Middle third: aortic arch to inferior pulmonary vein (50%)
3. Lower third: inferior pulmonary vein to gastro-oesophageal junction (20%)
   a. supra-diaphragmatic oesophagus
   b. intra-abdominal oesophagus

Spread of oesophageal carcinoma
1. Direct spread
   a. Submucosal spread in either a longitudinal or circumferential direction
   b. Transmural spread to adjacent structures:
      (i) mediastinal pleura
      (ii) lung
      (iii) aorta
      (iv) tracheo-bronchial tree
      (v) pericardium
      (vi) left recurrent laryngeal nerve
      (vii) diaphragmatic crura
2. Lymphatic spread
   a. Intramural lymphatic permeation and embolisation produce small microscopic metastases well beyond the macroscopic limits of tumour growth
   b. Regional lymphatic nodal metastases are dependent on the site of the oesophageal tumour.
      (i) Upper third – cervical nodes
      (ii) middle third – hilar, subcarinal and paratracheal nodes
      (iii) lower third – coeliac nodes
3. Blood-borne spread
   a. Liver
   b. Lungs
   c. Brain

Curative treatment of oesophageal carcinoma
1. Adenocarcinoma of the oesophagus is radioresistant and surgery offers the only hope of cure
2. Squamous oesophageal carcinoma is moderately radiosensitive; the size of the tumour and its degree of differentiation will determine the response to radiotherapy
3. The presence of intramural submucosal spread of tumour and its possible lymphatic permeation and embolisation require a 7.5–10 cm longitudinal clearance of normal oesophagus beyond the macroscopic limits of the tumour: the absence of

tumour at the resection margins can be confirmed by histological examination of frozen sections
4. Access to an adequate length of normal oesophagus dictates the surgical approach to oesophagectomy.
5. The pattern of lymphatic spread and the proximity of vital structures dictate that en bloc radical resection is feasible only for tumours arising in the lower third of the oesophagus

Treatment of tumours of the lower third
1. Thoraco-abdominal oesophago-gastrectomy with jejunal replacement
   a. Indicated for tumours below the diaphragm which are usually adenocarcinomas arising from the cardia of the stomach
   b. Left thoraco-abdominal incision allows radical excision of the stomach, spleen, tail of the pancreas, omentum and corresponding lymph nodes
   c. Continuity is restored by oesophago-jejunal anastomosis using a Roux loop
2. Two stage (Ivor Lewis) oesophago-gastrectomy with gastric replacement
   a. Indicated for tumours of the lower third above the diaphragmatic hiatus
   b. Laparotomy is performed and the stomach mobilised on the right gastric and right gastro-epiploic arteries
   c. The duodenum is mobilised by Kocherisation and a pyloromyotomy or pyloroplasty performed
   d. The abdomen is closed and the patient repositioned to allow a right thoracotomy
   e. Via the right pleural cavity the lower oesophagus is mobilised and the mobilised stomach drawn up into the chest
   f. The tumour is resected with an adequate clearance of macroscopically normal distal oesophagus and proximal stomach
   g. Continuity is restored by oesophago-gastric anastomosis

Treatment of tumours of the middle third
1. Ivor Lewis oesophagectomy with gastric replacement
   a. May be a suitable procedure for tumours in the distal half of the middle third
   b. For patients with tumours in the proximal half this operation involves a technically difficult anastomosis in the superior mediastinum; leakage from this anastomosis is associated with a high mortality
   c. Three stage total oesophagectomy provides a safer alternative as it avoids an intra-thoracic anastomosis

2. Three stage (McKeown) total oesophagectomy
   a. The stomach is mobilised via a laparotomy incision as in the Ivor Lewis procedure
   b. The thoracic oesophagus is mobilised via a right thoracotomy incision
   c. The cervical oesophagus is mobilised through a right supra-clavicular incision
   d. As an alternative to right thoracotomy the oesophagus may be mobilised by blind dissection via the abdominal and cervical incisions
   e. Following removal of the intra-thoracic and intra-abdominal portions of the oesophagus, the oesophago-gastric junction is closed and the gastric fundus anastomosed to the cervical oesophagus
   f. Anastomotic dehiscence leads to a cervical oesophageal fistula which will usually close spontaneously

Treatment of tumours of the upper third
1. Radiotherapy is often the treatment of choice
   a. With the introduction of megavoltage irradiation the results of radiotherapy have improved
   b. The high operative mortality of oesophagectomy is avoided
2. Three stage (McKeown) total oesophagectomy is an alternate to radiotherapy

Palliative treatment of unresectable oesophageal carcinoma
Relief of dysphagia is the main priority in treating inoperable tumours of the oesophagus
1. Surgical oesophageal intubation
   a. A laparotomy is performed and via a gastrotomy one of the various tubes, e.g. Mousseau–Barbin, Celestin is inserted by a pull-through technique
   b. Post-operative wound infection is very common and overall there is a high operative mortality
   c. The main complications related to the oesophageal tube are bolus obstruction, displacement of the prosthesis and gastro-oesophageal reflux
   d. Erosion of the oesophageal wall may later lead to perforation or formation of a fistula connecting with the tracheo-bronchial tree
2. Endoscopic oesophageal intubation
   a. The morbidity and mortality of this technique are much less than that of surgical intubation
   b. It can be performed using either a rigid or flexible endoscope
   c. The malignant stricture is visualised and a guide-wire passed through it

    d. Following dilatation the neoplasm is intubated with a silastic rubber tube using a Nottingham introducer

    e. Oesophageal perforation is the main complication of endoscopic dilatation and intubation occurring in up to 10% of patients

3. Oesophageal bypass

    a. Retrosternal or subcutaneous bypass of unresectable carcinomas using stomach, jejunum or colon has been reported

    b. Operative mortality is high and survival following surgery is short

    c. Most survivors are able to eat a normal diet

4. Radiotherapy

5. Laser (photodynamic) recanalisation

FURTHER READING

Earlam R, Cunha-Melo J R 1980 Oesophageal squamous cell carcinoma. A critical review of surgery. Br J Surg 67: 381–390

Earlam R, Cunha-Melo J R 1980 Oesophageal squamous cell carcinoma. A critical review of radiotherapy. Br J Surg 67: 457–461

Earlam R, Cunha-Melo J R 1982 Malignant oesophageal strictures: a review of techniques for palliative intubation. Br J Surg 69: 61–68

Hennessy T P J, O'Connell R 1984 Surgical treatment of squamous cell carcinoma of the oesophagus. Br J Surg 71: 750–751

McKeown K C 1987 Adventures on a surgical Everest. Eur J Surg Oncol 13: 375–398

Ogilvie A L, Dronfield M W, Ferguson R, Atkinson M 1982 Palliative intubation of oesophagogastric neoplasms at fibreoptic endoscopy. Gut 23: 1060–1067

Orringer M B 1983 Palliative procedures for oesophageal cancer. Surg Clin N Am 63: 941–950

DUODENAL ULCERATION

Objectives of treatment

1. Relieve symptoms
2. Heal ulcer
3. Prevent complications
4. Prevent recurrent ulceration

Medical treatment

1. Antacids

    a. Agents such as magnesium trisilicate, magnesium hydroxide, aluminium hydroxide and aluminium carbonate are frequently used for symptomatic relief of dyspepsia

    b. Large doses of antacids at frequent intervals are usually required to obtain healing in addition to symptomatic relief; for this reason compliance is often unsatisfactory

   c. Use of antacids alone will produce healing of duodenal ulcers in about 80% of patients within 4 weeks

   d. Constipation or diarrhoea are often significant

2. Coating agents

   a. Sucralfate (Antepsin), a basic aluminium salt of sulphated sucrose, forms a protective coat which adheres selectively to ulcerated areas and acts as a barrier to acid diffusion

   b. Tri-potassium di-citrato bismuthate (De-Nol) chelates with proteins at acid pHs forming a protective layer over the ulcer and heals duodenal ulcers at a similar rate to cimetidine

3. Carbenoxolone

   a. Carbenoxolone (Duogastrone), a licorice derivative, which acts by increasing the production, viscosity and glycoprotein content of mucus

   b. May cause salt and water retention, hypokalaemia and hypertension and its use is contra-indicated in those patients with cardiac disease, renal or hepatic insufficiency

4. H_2-receptor antagonists

   a. Cimetidine (Tagamet) and ranitidine (Zantac) are potent inhibitors of gastric acid secretion mediated via H_2 histamine receptors

   b. The rate of healing of peptic ulcers is similar for the two drugs; in most series up to 90% of duodenal ulcers are healed by an 8-week course of treatment

   c. Both drugs are tolerated well with a low incidence of side effects

   d. Skin rashes, headache and lethargy are the most commonly reported side effects

   e. More serious side effects include gynaecomastia and impotence in men, confusional states and hepatic dysfunction

5. Synthetic prostaglandin analogues

   a. Prostaglandins of the E series are cytoprotective, increasing both mucus and bicarbonate secretion

   b. In addition they inhibit gastric acid secretion

   c. Misoprostol, a PG_{E1} methylanalogue, has been shown to be as effective as cimetidine in healing duodenal ulcers

   d. Diarrhoea is an important side effect occurring in up to one third of patients

6. Substituted benzimidazole compounds

   a. Gastric acid production is reduced by inhibition of the hydrogen-potassium ATPase enzyme which normally drives the proton pump mechanism of the parietal cells

   b. Omeprazole produces a marked reduction in gastric acid secretion and is undergoing clinical trials

Indications for surgical treatment

The improved efficiency and safety of medical treatment,

particularly the introduction of H_2-receptor antagonists in 1976, have greatly reduced the number of surgical operations for duodenal ulceration. Operative treatment is indicated in the following situations.

1. Failure of symptomatic control and ulcer healing despite adequate medical treatment.
2. Recurrent ulceration
3. Complicated duodenal ulcer
   a. Haemorrhage
   b. Perforation
   c. Gastric outflow obstruction

Operative treatment of uncomplicated chronic duodenal ulceration
The ideal elective surgical treatment for chronic duodenal ulceration should have the following characteristics:
   a. low operative mortality
   b. low incidence of recurrent peptic ulceration
   c. low incidence of post-gastric surgical syndromes
1. Highly selective vagotomy (HSV) (Parietal cell or proximal gastric vagotomy)
   a. Only the acid secretory cell mass within the body of the stomach is denervated
   b. Innervation of the antro-pyloro-duodenal segment is preserved via the anterior and posterior nerves of Latarjet which are left intact thus obviating the need for a gastric drainage procedure
   c. Avascular necrosis of the lesser curve is a rare complication occurring in 0.2% of all patients but is associated with a high mortality rate
   d. Overall mortality in experienced hands is less than 0.5%
   e. A technically inadequate HSV, usually due to operative difficulties, is responsible for those patients who are Hollander positive immediately after the first post-operative week; these patients are at risk of recurrent ulceration
   f. Partial vagal reinnervation of the lesser curve occurs in over 50% of patients whose Hollander status becomes positive having been negative at the end of the first post-operative week; peak acid output is only a fraction of its pre-operative value and a late positive result has no value in predicting future recurrence of the ulcer
   g. The rate of recurrent ulceration after HSV continues to increase with length of follow-up
   h. Enthusiasts of the operation claim recurrence rates of 2–5% after 5–8 years
   i. Dumping and diarrhoea are rarely seen after highly selective vagotomy
2. Posterior truncal vagotomy and anterior lesser curve seromyotomy

   a. Technically an easier operation than highly selective
      vagotomy and requiring only half the operating time
   b. Seromyotomy can be performed using a stapling device
      which further reduces operating time
   c. Very safe operation in which the risks of lesser curve
      necrosis are abolished
   d. Recurrence rates are similar to those of HSV
   e. As with HSV dumping and diarrhoea are both very rare
      complications
3. Selective gastric vagotomy and drainage
   a. Hepatic branches of the anterior vagus and the coeliac
      branches of the posterior vagus are preserved
   b. Recurrence rates are similar to those of truncal vagotomy
   c. Severe dumping occurs in 10% of patients and diarrhoea in
      15%
   d. This procedure has failed to become a popular alternative to
      truncal vagotomy and drainage because the complication
      rates were not significantly reduced
4. Truncal vagotomy and drainage
   a. After 40 years this remains the most commonly performed
      operation for chronic duodenal ulceration.
   b. Relatively simple operation which is quick to perform
   c. Operative mortality rate is less than 1%
   d. Recurrences are seen in up to 5–10% of cases
   e. Significant dumping is seen in 25% of cases and diarrhoea
      in 20–25%
5. Truncal vagotomy and antrectomy
   a. Reduces gastric acid output by over 90% and provides the
      most effective safeguard against recurrent ulceration, most
      series showing recurrence rates of 0.5–1%
   b. Operative mortality is 1–2%
   c. Dumping occurs in 25% of patients and significant diarrhoea
      in 10%
   d. Although practised widely by some surgeons, especially
      those in the USA, gastric resection should normally be
      reserved for those patients with recurrent ulceration

Complications of duodenal ulceration and their management
1. Perforation
   a. Overall incidence of perforated peptic ulcer is declining
   b. Male: female ratio is falling owing to a decline in the
      incidence of the condition in men and an increased
      incidence in women
   c. Average mortality is 10–15%, being higher in elderly
      patients and in those where there is excessive delay
      between perforation and surgical intervention
   d. Simple closure of the perforation incorporating an omental
      patch and combined with peritoneal lavage is followed by a

2-month course of H_2-receptor antagonists in those patients
without a long previous history of ulcer dyspepsia
   e. Patients with a long dyspeptic history and not previously
      treated with H_2-receptor antagonists are also treated in a
      similar fashion; those with recurrent symptoms in whom
      the ulcer fails to heal despite prolonged medical treatment
      should then be considered for definitive surgical treatment
      at a later stage
   f. Definitive treatment of an apparently chronic ulcer at the
      time of perforation should be reserved for those patients
      who perforate while taking H_2-receptor antagonists or who
      have suffered other complications. Provided the surgeon is
      expert and there is no excessive delay between perforation
      and laparotomy definitive surgery can be performed without
      increased operative mortality
2. Haemorrhage
   a. In many patients haemorrhage stops spontaneously; only
      those patients with continued or repeated haemorrhage will
      require surgical treatment
   b. Despite improved diagnostic techniques and attempts at
      better selection for operative treatment the overall operative
      mortality is still approximately 10%
   c. Risk factors include advanced age, profuse haemorrhage,
      hypotensive shock and chronic ulceration
   d. There is no convincing evidence that H_2-receptor
      antagonists are of benefit in treating acute haemorrhage
      from a duodenal ulcer
   e. Surgical treatment normally consists of truncal vagotomy,
      pyloro-duodenotomy, under-running the bleeding vessel
      and ulcer with a non-absorbable suture and pyloroplasty
   f. In the presence of severe duodenal scarring pyloroplasty
      may not be possible; in these cases the duodenotomy is
      closed longitudinally and a gastro-enterostomy fashioned
   g. Highly selective vagotomy with a duodenotomy is an
      alternative procedure which preserves the pylorus and
      avoids the complications of vagotomy; the bleeding vessel
      is under-run and the duodenum closed longitudinally
   h. A Polya gastrectomy will eliminate the risk of further
      haemorrhage from the ulcer in the post-operative period
   i. As an alternative to operative treatment various endoscopic
      treatments such as laser photocoagulation, bipolar
      diathermy coagulation, heat probes and ethanol injection
      continue to be evaluated
3. Gastric outflow obstruction ('pyloric stenosis')
   a. Truncal or selective vagotomy and drainage is probably the
      most favoured technique; gastro-jejunostomy is required in
      cases of severe duodenal scarring
   b. Partial gastrectomy with gastro-jejunal anastomosis (Polya

gastrectomy) may be required as a secondary procedure in those cases with gastric stasis following vagotomy
  c. Highly selective vagotomy accompanied by duodenoplasty or digital dilatation of the stenosed segment through a small gastrotomy in the denervated area of the stomach avoids post-vagotomy or post-gastrectomy syndromes and in expert hands can be performed with minimal risk of further stenosis

FURTHER READING

Editorial 1986 Peptic ulcer: which patients to consider for surgery. Drug Therap Bull 24: 77–78
Murray W R 1986 Surgical management of haemorrhage from peptic ulceration. Br J Surg 73: 947–948
Raimes S A, Devlin H B 1987 Perforated duodenal ulcer. Br J Surg 74: 81–82
Simpson C J, Lamont G, Macdonald I, Smith I S 1987 Effect of cimetidine on prognosis after simple closure of perforated duodenal ulcer. Br J Surg 74: 104–105
Taylor T V 1985 Vagotomy and peptic ulceration – an update. In: Taylor I (ed) Progress in Surgery Vol 1 Churchill Livingstone, Edinburgh pp 52–66
Watkins R M, Dennison A R, Collin J 1984 What has happened to perforated peptic ulcer? Br J Surg 71: 774–778

COMPLICATIONS OF GASTRIC SURGERY

In addition to the complications which may follow any laparotomy several specific complications may occur after gastric surgery especially gastrectomy.

Haemorrhage

Aetiological factors
  1. Intra-peritoneal haemorrhage
      a. Torn splenic capsule
      b. Insecure ligatures on major vascular pedicles or omental vessels
      c. Haemorrhagic diathesis
  2. Intra-luminal haemorrhage
      a. Suture line haemorrhage
      b. Haemorrhage from duodenal ulcer previously under-run or ulcer in gastric remnant not previously noted
      c. Acute erosions of gastric mucosa
      d. Oesophageal varices
      e. Haemorrhagic diathesis

Treatment
  1. Blood transfusion
  2. Naso-gastric aspiration
  3. Operative treatment

Acute gastric (remnant) dilatation

Large fluid and electrolyte losses may occur with consequent hypovolaemic shock. Gross distension of the stomach or gastric remnant may cause disruption of the suture line

Prevention
1. Maintenance of fluid and electrolyte balance
2. Continued naso-gastric aspiration until post-operative paralytic ileus has resolved

Treatment
1. Naso-gastric aspiration
2. Correction of fluid and electrolyte imbalance

Acute pancreatitis

Although a rare condition, acute pancreatitis following gastric surgery is associated with a high mortality which is often greater than 50%

Aetiological factors
1. Pancreatic trauma during mobilisation of a posterior penetrating duodenal or gastric ulcer.
2. Duct of Santorini (accessory pancreatic duct) may be injured in transfixing and ligating the pancreato-duodenal artery.
3. Pancreatic tail is resected in radical gastrectomy
4. Post-gastrectomy pancreatitis may follow mobilisation of the stomach and duodenum and occur without any apparent pancreatic trauma

Treatment
Refer to Pages 35–38

Duodenal stump leakage and fistula ('blow out')

An infrequent but very serious and sometimes fatal complication of Polya gastrectomy with a maximal incidence on the 4th and 5th post-operative days.

Aetiological factors
1. Afferent loop obstruction
2. Difficult closure of the duodenal stump especially if a large oedematous ulcer is penetrating the head of the pancreas
3. Extensive mobilisation of the first part of the duodenum causing ischaemic necrosis

Prevention
1. Careful closure of the duodenal stump
2. Ensure adequate drainage of afferent loop

Treatment
1. Immediate and adequate drainage of bile, pancreatic and duodenal secretions preferably by sump drainage to protect the surrounding skin
2. Maintenance of fluid and electrolyte balance
3. Total parenteral nutrition (TPN): Refer to Pages 243–248
4. If the afferent loop is draining freely spontaneous closure should occur

Anastomotic leakage

Aetiological factors
1. Poor surgical technique
2. Gastric (remnant) dilatation
3. Malnutrition
4. Ischaemia of suture line; if splenectomy is required division of the short gastric vessels may render the gastric remnant ischaemic

Treatment
1. Immediate and adequate drainage with closure of the anastomotic dehiscence where possible
2. Rarely an ischaemic gastric remnant will require excision and reconstruction using a Roux loop of jejunum
3. Maintenance of fluid and electrolyte balance
4. Total parenteral nutrition while awaiting spontaneous closure of any gastric fistula

Afferent loop obstruction

This is a rare but serious complication of Polya gastrectomy which usually occurs in the first few post-operative days and may cause early duodenal stump leakage. It usually presents with acute epigastric pain associated with the absence of bile in the gastric aspirates. An elevated serum amylase suggests the diagnosis

Aetiological factors
1. Stomal oedema
2. Twisting or kinking of a long afferent loop
3. Narrowing of afferent loop by sutures used to create the gastro-jejunostomy

Treatment
1. Urgent surgical intervention is required and the gastrectomy revised to provide an adequate stoma shortening the afferent loop if necessary
2. An entero-enterostomy between the afferent and efferent loops is an alternative manoeuvre

Afferent loop (bilious vomiting) syndrome

This syndrome may occur after gastro-enterostomy or Polya gastrectomy. Typically the patient presents with intermittent right hypochondrial pain with associated distension and nausea which are are relieved by vomiting bile-stained fluid. The afferent loop fails to empty when food is present in the stomach, becomes gradually more distended with pancreatic and biliary secretions and finally empties into the gastric remnant when the food has passed into the efferent loop.

Treatment
1. The afferent loop is shortened to improve its drainage
2. Conversion to a Roux-en Y anastomosis is an alternative

Efferent loop obstruction

Any delay in gastric emptying causes excessive nasogastric aspirates.

Aetiological factors
1. Stomal oedema or stenosis
2. Retrograde jejuno-gastric intussusception

Treatment
1. Maintenance of fluid and electrolyte balance
2. Total parenteral nutrition may be required if delayed gastric emptying is persistent
3. If a jejuno-gastric intussusception does not reduce spontaneously operative treatment is required

Small intestinal obstruction

Aetiological factors
1. Following Polya gastrectomy with a retrocolic gastro-jejunal anastomosis a loop of small intestine can pass through the defect produced in the transverse mesocolon: this is prevented by closing the defect by suturing its edges to the gastric remnant so that the anastomosis lies entirely in the infracolic compartment
2. Following an antecolic Polya gastrectomy a loop of small intestine (Stammers' loop) can pass between the gastro-jejunal anastomosis anteriorly and the transverse colon posteriorly: this can be prevented by suturing the anastomosis to the transverse mesocolon.
3. Bolus obstruction of the small intestine

Treatment
1. Replacement of fluid and electrolyte losses
2. Naso-gastric aspiration
3. Operative correction of small intestinal obstruction

Subphrenic and subhepatic abscess

Aetiological factors
1. Perforated peptic ulcer
2. Duodenal stump leakage
3. Anastomotic leakage
4. Intra-peritoneal haemorrhage
5. Splenectomy

Treatment
1. Percutaneous aspiration under ultrasound or computed tomographic guidance
2. Operative exploration and drainage

Recurrent peptic ulceration
Refer to Pages 13–14

Anastomotic (stomal) ulceration
Stomal ulceration can occur after any operation in which gastric and jejunal mucosa become continuous. The highest incidence was seen after simple gastro-jejunostomy for duodenal ulcer. Typically a stomal ulcer is now found at the origin of the efferent loop after a Polya gastrectomy and it often presents with epigastric pain. Fibreoptic gastroscopy provides the most reliable means of confirming the diagnosis. Complications include perforation, haemorrhage, stomal obstruction and gastro-jejuno-colic fistula.

Aetiological factors
1. Incomplete vagotomy
2. Inadequate gastric resection
3. Hypergastrinaemia (Zollinger–Ellison syndrome)
   Refer to Pages 196–198
4. Ulcerogenic drugs

Treatment
1. Supra-diaphragmatic truncal vagotomy may be performed through a left thoracotomy incision in those patients who have previously had an incomplete vagotomy and now have an uncomplicated stomal ulcer
2. Patients with inadequate gastric resections and complete vagotomy require revision of their gastrectomy
3. All complicated stomal ulcers should be assessed at laparotomy
4. Distortion and stenosis of a gastro-jejunal anastomosis require revision gastrectomy in which the stomal ulcer is resected along with the adjacent stomach and a new gastro-jejunal anastomosis is fashioned. (An end-to-end jejuno-jejunal anastomosis between the original ends of the afferent and efferent loops will be sited either on the new afferent or

efferent loop depending on the length of the original afferent loop.)

5. Haemorrhage can often be controlled by gastro-jejunotomy and underrunning the stomal ulcer although further gastric resection or vagotomy is required to prevent further bleeding
6. Peforation of a stomal ulcer is treated by simple closure followed by gastric resection or vagotomy
7. A gastro-jejuno-colic fistula is resected along with part of the stomach, its opening into the colon closed and a new ante-colic gastro-jejunostomy fashioned. (In patients with poor general condition a staged resection (Pfeiffer's operation) is safer.)

Post-cibal syndromes

(A) Early dumping
Patients experience weakness and dizziness often accompanied by palpitations, and sweating. Symptoms occur during or soon after a meal and are relieved by lying down. Examination reveals a tachycardia, hypotension and pallor.

Mechanism
1. Rapid emptying of hyperosmolor gastric contents into the jejunum draws extracellular fluid into the intestinal lumen
2. The consequent reduction in plasma volume is indicated by an increased haematocrit

Treatment
1. Eat meals slowly and avoid foods known to precipitate symptoms
2. Take fluids and solid food separately
3. Low-carbohydrate, high-fibre diet
4. Lie down after meals
5. Reversed (anti-peristaltic) jejunal segment

(B) Late dumping (reactive hypoglycaemia)
Weakness, tremor, palpitations and sweating occur about 2 hours after a meal. Loss of consciousness may occur.

Mechanism
1. Rapid absorption of carbohydrate by the small intestine produces dramatic rise in blood sugar followed by secretion of large quantities of insulin
2. Increased plasma insulin levels produce a period of hypoglycaemia which may be profound

Treatment
1. Tolbutamide 500 mg before each meal
2. Low-carbohydrate, high-fibre diet
3. Oral glucose to be taken if hypoglycaemic symptoms occur
4. Reversed (anti-peristaltic) jejunal segment

Diarrhoea
Diarrhoea following gastric surgery is usually episodic but in some cases may be continuous. It is more common after truncal vagotomy than after gastrectomy.

Mechanisms
1. Rapid gastric emptying
2. Vagal denervation of small intestine
3. Underlying small intestinal pathology, e.g. coeliac disease, alactasia

Treatment
1. Anti-diarrhoeal agents e.g. codeine phosphate 30–60 mg 4-hourly
2. Avoid any aggravating foods
3. Reversed (anti-peristaltic) jejunal segment

Nutritional disturbances

(A) Weight loss
Weight loss is seen to some extent after most gastric operations and in almost all cases undergoing total gastrectomy.

Mechanisms
1. Reduced dietary intake
2. Impaired intestinal absorption

(B) Osteomalacia
Clinically significant osteomalacia is a relatively uncommon complication of gastrectomy but a subclinical form occurs in 15–20% of patients.

Mechanism – Malabsorption of vitamin D

Treatment – Vitamin D and oral calcium supplementation

(C) Anaemia
Although often mild, iron deficiency anaemia occurs in up to 50% of patients following gastric surgery. Vitamin B_{12} deficiency is inevitable after total gastric surgery unless prophylactic parenteral therapy is given.

Mechanisms
1. Reduction of gastric acid impairs iron absorption as ferrous salts are more readily absorbed than their ferric counterparts
2. Iron deficiency is especially liable to occur if the duodenum has been bypassed as it is an important site for iron absorption
3. Vitamin B_{12} (cyanocobalamin) deficiency occurs after total gastrectomy due to lack of intrinsic factor normally secreted by the cells of the body and fundus of the stomach

Treatment
1. Oral iron supplementation
2. Regular parenteral vitamin B_{12} therapy

Gastric carcinoma

There is an increased incidence of gastric carcinoma following most forms of gastric surgery. In most cases there is a delay of 15–25 years between the original surgery and the development of a carcinoma. Bacterial colonisation of the hypochlorhydric stomach may have a direct or indirect carcinogenic effect. The overall risk of developing a gastric carcinoma after gastric surgery is quite small and regular endoscopic screening of patients after gastric surgery is not at present cost-effective. Identification of high risk groups is still required.

FURTHER READING

Clark C G, Fresini A, Gledhill T 1985 Cancer following gastric surgery. Br J Surg 72: 591–594

Cuschieri A 1977 Isoperistaltic and antiperistaltic jejunal interposition for the dumping syndrome. A comparative study. J R Coll Surg Edin 22: 319–324

Mackie C R, Hall A W, Clark J, Wisbey M, Baker P R, Cuschieri A 1981 The effect of isoperistaltic jejunal interposition upon gastric emptying. Surg Gynecol Obstet 153: 813–819

Sawyers J L, Herrington J L 1973 Superiority of antiperistaltic jejunal segments in management of severe dumping symptoms. Ann Surg 178: 311–321

Hepato-biliary surgery

INVESTIGATION AND MANAGEMENT OF THE JAUNDICED PATIENT

Classification
1. Pre-hepatic jaundice
   a. Haemolytic anaemias
   b. Familial non-haemolytic hyperbilirubinaemia
      (i) Gilbert's syndrome
      (ii) Crigler–Najjar syndrome
      (iii) Dubin–Johnson syndrome
      (iv) Rotor's syndrome
2. Hepatic jaundice
   a. Acute viral hepatitis e.g. hepatitis-A, hepatitis-B, Non-A non-B hepatitis, infectious mononucleosis
   b. Cirrhosis, e.g. alcoholic, cryptogenic, primary biliary, Wilson's disease, haemochromatosis, α_1-anti-trypsin deficiency
   c. Chronic active hepatitis
   d. Drugs, e.g. halothane, chlorpromazine, norethisterone
   e. Hepatic toxins, e.g. alcohol, carbon tetrachloride, vinyl chloride, paracetamol
   f. Hepatic tumours, e.g. hepatoma, secondary carcinoma
   g. Liver abscess
   h. Parasitic infestations, e.g. hydatid disease, Weil's disease
3. Post-hepatic jaundice
   a. Choledocholithiasis
   b. Traumatic bile duct stricture
   c. Biliary atresia
   d. Bile duct carcinoma (cholangiocarcinoma)
   e. Carcinoma of gall bladder
   f. Enlarged lymph nodes in porta hepatis
   g. Sclerosing cholangitis
   h. Pancreatic carcinoma
   i. Pancreatitis
   j. Carcinoma of ampulla of Vater

Differential diagnosis

	Pre-hepatic jaundice	Hepatic jaundice	Post-hepatic jaundice
History			
	Family history	Recent contacts with hepatitis patients	Dark urine and pale stools
		Foreign travel	Pruritus
		Anorexia, malaise	Abdominal pain (biliary calculi)
		Cigarette aversion (acute hepatitis)	Fever, sweating and rigors (cholangitis)
		Alcohol or drug abuse	Weight loss and anorexia (pancreatic carcinoma)
		Hepatotoxic drugs	Previous biliary surgery (traumatic biliary stricture)
		Blood transfusion	
		Homosexual practice	
		Tatooing	
Clinical examination			
	Mild icterus	Hepatomegaly	Hepatomegaly
		Signs of chronic parenchymal liver disease	Palpable gall bladder (Courvoisier's sign)
		Signs of liver failure	Signs of advanced malignant disease
		Signs of portal hypertension	
		Venepuncture marks	
Urinalysis			
Bilirubin	−	±	+
Urobilinogen	+	↑	−
Serum analysis			
Bilirubin:			
unconjugated	↑ ↑	↑	Normal
conjugated	Normal	↑	↑ ↑
Transaminases	Normal	↑ ↑ ↑	Normal or ↑
Alkaline phosphatase	Normal	Normal or ↑	↑ ↑ ↑
γ-glutamyl trans- peptidase	Normal	↑ (alcoholic liver disease)	Normal
Prothrombin time	Normal	Normal or ↑ (poor correction with vitamin K)	↑ (good correction with vitamin K)
Albumin	Normal	Normal or ↓	Normal

Differential diagnosis
For the surgeon, there are two basic problems in the investigation
of the jaundiced patient:
 1. Rapid differentation between 'medical' and 'surgical' causes of
    jaundice
    a. Unnecessary or poorly timed surgery on patients with
       cirrhosis or hepatitis is associated with an increased
       morbidity and mortality
    b. The morbidity and mortality of surgery in patients with
       obstructive jaundice is related to the severity and duration
       of the jaundice; early surgery in these cases is therefore
       important
 2. For 'surgical' causes determination of the site, nature and
    extent of the obstructing lesion
Cases of pre-hepatic jaundice are usually obvious and the main
diagnostic difficulty is differentiating between hepatic and post-
hepatic or obstructive causes. The history, clinical examination and
certain basic investigations are of great importance. Refer to Page 25

Important special investigations
 1. Abdominal ultrasonography
    a. Easily performed, rapid and non-invasive test
    b. Distinguishes hepato-cellular jaundice from jaundice due to
       extra-hepatic obstruction with an accuracy of over 80%
    c. The site and cause of extra-hepatic biliary obstruction is not
       always shown: gallstones at the lower end of the common
       bile duct are frequently not visualised with ultrasonography
       and the head of the pancreas may be obscured by intestinal
       gas
    d. If the biliary tree is dilated and if further information about
       the nature, site and extent of the obstructing lesion is
       required, either endoscopic retrograde cholangio-
       pancreatography (ERCP) or percutaneous trans-hepatic
       cholangiography (PTC) can be performed
    e. If the biliary tree is not dilated percutaneous liver biopsy
       should be performed provided any coagulation defects can
       be corrected
 2. Percutaneous liver biopsy
    a. Performed if the bile ducts are not dilated after any
       coagulation defects have been corrected
    b. Histological examination of biopsy material should reveal
       the nature and aetiology of the hepato-cellular defect
 3. Endoscopic retrograde cholangio-pancreatography (ERCP)
    a. Morbidity and mortality rates are similar to those of
       percutaneous trans-hepatic cholangiography
    b. Can be performed in the presence of mild coagulation
       defects
    c. ERCP is used in preference to percutaneous trans-hepatic

cholangiography for choledocholithiasis, sclerosing
cholangitis and pancreatic diseases
d. Therapeutic manoeuvres can be performed in some cases.
Refer to Page 32
4. Percutaneous trans-hepatic cholangiography (PTC)
a. An intra-hepatic biliary radical is punctured and contrast
injected under radiographic control to outline the dilated
biliary tree
b. The high risk of biliary peritonitis associated with use of
wide sheathed needles has been reduced following the
introduction of the finer skiny needle
c. Success rate is related to the degree of intra-hepatic bile
duct dilatation and the number of needle passes into the
liver: up to 12 passes are required to achieve a success rate
of 99%
d. Contra-indicated in the presence of ascites or coagulation
defects
e. Complications which include cholangitis, haemorrhage and
bile leakage occur in less than 5% of patients
f. Facilities for urgent laparotomy should always be available
5. Computed tomography (CT)
a. Demonstrates dilated bile ducts in 80–90% of cases
b. Useful in defining space-occupying lesions within the liver
and certain extra-hepatic lesions notably lymphomas and
pancreatic neoplasms
c. Unlikely to replace the need for ERCP and PTC

Pre-operative management of the jaundiced patient
1. Correct and maintain fluid and electrolyte balance
2. Nutritional support
3. Correct haemorrhagic diathesis
a. Vitamin K given by intra-venous injection
b. Fresh frozen plasma
c. Platelet concentrates
4. Intra-venous mannitol to prevent acute oliguric renal failure
5. Bile salts
a. Obstructive jaundice is associated with disruption of the
normal entero-hepatic circulation of bile salts
b. Endotoxaemia and subsequent renal failure may be caused
by increased endotoxin absorption from the intestine which
is the result of a deficiency of intra-luminal bile salts
c. This deficiency can be corrected by oral administration of
bile salts
d. Various studies have suggested that bile salts such as
sodium deoxycholate can prevent post-operative renal
failure in jaundiced patients
6. Prophylactic antibiotics
a. The intra-venous route of administration is favoured as it

provides high serum levels of antibiotic at the time of
surgery
  b. A broad-spectrum penicillin such as mezlocillin, piperacillin
     or ticarcillin or alternatively third-generation cephalosporin
     such as cefuroxime, or cephamandole are examples of
     suitable prophylactic agents
  c. Aminoglycosides should not be used routinely but reserved
     for serious infections such as ascending cholangitis
7. Percutaneous trans-hepatic biliary drainage
  a. The obstructed biliary tree is catheterised percutaneously
     with a pigtail catheter at the time of fine needle trans-
     hepatic cholangiography
  b. Free drainage of bile for up to three weeks prior to definitive
     surgery is associated with a reduction in serum bilirubin
     level
  c. Controlled clinical trials have shown no reduction in
     mortality using pre-operative percutaneous biliary drainage
     in patients with malignant biliary obstruction
  d. Complications include sepsis, tube dislodgement, bile
     peritonitis, haemobilia and biliary fistulae
  e. Closed systems of external biliary drainage prevent
     exogenous bacterial contamination
8. Endoscopic biliary drainage
  a. Endoscopic sphincterotomy is indicated in patients with
     ascending cholangitis secondary to calculous obstruction of
     the biliary tract
  b. Especially in elderly patients this procedure reduces the
     mortality associated with emergency surgery: Refer to Page
     32

Surgical management
This will depend on the exact nature of the pathology causing the
obstructive jaundice.
1. Choledocholithiasis
  a. Primary common bile duct stones are normally removed via
     a longitudinal supra-duodenal choledochotomy
  b. Biliary calculi can be extracted from the duct using
     Desjardin's forceps or a biliary Fogarty catheter; it may be
     possible to flush small calculi into the duodenum
  c. A trans-duodenal sphincterotomy may be necessary to
     remove stones impacted at the lower end of the common
     bile duct
  d. Alternative drainage procedures such as
     choledochoduodenostomy may be indicated in poor risk
     elderly patients where the common bile duct is significantly
     dilated
  e. Retained common bile duct stones: Refer to Pages 49–53

2. Bile duct carcinoma (cholangiocarcinoma)
   a. This slow growing scirrhous tumour usually presents with obstructive jaundice
   b. Most tumours occur at or near the hilum of the liver making curative resection technically difficult
   c. In a minority of patients with hilar lesions complete excision is possible although considerable hepatic resection may be required: biliary drainage is via a hepatico-jejunostomy using a Roux loop
   d. Many lesions are inoperable due to invasion of the hepatic portal vein or hepatic artery
   e. Palliative treatment involves dilatation of the strictured bile duct at operation followed by intubation
   f. In patients who present a high operative risk intubation can be performed via the percutaneous transhepatic route and may be combined with radiotherapy using ^{192}Ir irridium wires
   g. Orthotopic liver allotransplantation should be offered to young patients with otherwise unresectable tumours provided there is no evidence of distant metastases
   h. Lesions of the common bile duct if operable are best treated by Whipple's procedure
3. Traumatic bile duct stricture
   a. The majority of post-operative bile duct strictures follow biliary tract surgery
   b. Iatrogenic bile duct strictures complicate 1 in 500–600 biliary tract operations; in over 90% this is cholecystectomy
   c. Patients usually present with obstructive jaundice often with intermittent cholangitis
   d. Biliary stasis encourages stone formation and if untreated secondary biliary cirrhosis soon occurs
   e. Most strictures involve the common hepatic duct and are usually repaired by hepaticodocho-jejunostomy using a Roux loop
   f. For higher strictures the hepatic plate is dissected to expose the right and left hepatic ducts; if the two ducts are separated by fibrous tissue with no communication between them hepatico-jejunostomy will involve two anastomoses to the same Roux loop
   g. Strictures of the common bile duct are less common and can usually be treated by choledocho-duodenostomy or choledocho-jejunostomy using a Roux loop
   h. Identification of the injured bile duct and the proximal dilated ducts is aided by intra-operative cholangiography
   i. Once the proximal ducts have been indentified any stones or biliary sludge should be removed

    j. Establishing mucosal continuity between the biliary and digestive tracts is an important factor in preventing subsequent stricture formation

    k. A stent is usually used to facilitate and splint the biliary–enteric anastomosis

4. Pancreatic carcinoma
    Refer to Pages 45–47

5. Carcinoma of ampulla of Vater
    a. Pancreatico-duodenectomy (Whipple's operation) performed as a one stage procedure is the surgical treatment of choice
    b. Operative mortality should be less than 10%
    c. Choledocho-jejunostomy or cholecysto-jejunostomy are useful palliative procedures in patients with inoperable tumours
    d. Patients who are deemed unfit for surgery may be treated by endoscopic sphincterotomy or placement of an endoprosthesis

6. Acute pancreatitis
    Refer to Pages 35–36

7. Chronic pancreatitis
    Refer to Pages 41–42

8. Biliary atresia
    a. Approximately 10% of all cases of biliary atresia can be treated by choledocho-jejunostomy using a Roux loop
    b. The majority of infants with biliary atresia have no patent extra-hepatic bile ducts; surgical treatment in these cases comprises hepatic porto-enterostomy (Kasai operation)

Aetiology of post-operative jaundice

1. Increased bilirubin production
    a. Blood transfusion especially stored blood or blood which has been mis-matched
    b. Reabsorption of post-operative haematomas.

2. Hepato-cellular damage
    a. Hypovolaemic shock
    b. Cardiac failure
    c. Exacerbation of pre-existing liver disease
    d. Halothane hepatitis
    e. Other hepatotoxic drugs
    f. Viral hepatitis
    g. Severe sepsis

3. Extra-hepatic obstruction
    a. Residual bile duct calculi
    b. Bile duct trauma
    c. Pancreatitis

The most severe form of post-operative jaundice is caused by halothane hepatitis. This is a rare condition which tends to occur after repeated halothane exposures especially when the interval between each anaesthetic is short. Elderly, obese females are particularly at risk. The condition is characterised by a pyrexia with rigors which usually occur about 7 days after the first exposure to halothane. There are often other non-specific symptoms and right hypochondrial pain. Jaundice occurs after a further 2–3 days. The serum transaminase levels are elevated. After several exposures to halothane the condition may occur any time after the first post-operative day. The overall mortality is approximately 50% and is increased in those patients with severe jaundice.

FURTHER READING

Cahill C J 1983 Prevention of postoperative renal failure in patients with obstructive jaundice – the role of bile salts. Br J Surg 70: 590–595
Collins P G, Gorey T F 1984 Iatrogenic biliary stricture: presentation and management. Br J Surg 71: 980–982
Johnson A G, Hosking S W 1987 Appraisal of the management of bile duct stones. Br J Surg 74: 555–560
Lai E C S, Tomkins R K, Roslyn J J, Mann L L 1987 Proximal bile duct cancer: Quality of survival. Ann Surg 205: 111–118
Lokich J J, Kane R A, Harrison D A, McDermott W V 1987 Biliary tract obstruction secondary to cancer: management guidelines and selected literature review: J Clin Oncol 5: 969–981
Sherlock S 1981 Diseases of the Liver and Biliary system, 6th edition, Blackwell Scientific Publications Oxford
Warnes T W 1982 Investigation of the jaundiced patient. Br J Hosp Med 28: 385–391

ENDOSCOPIC RETROGRADE CHOLANGIO-PANCREATOGRAPHY (ERCP)

Technique
1. Performed by an experienced endoscopist using side-viewing duodenoscope
2. Full oesophago-gastro-duodenoscopy is carefully performed to exclude any associated abnormalities
3. Success rate and number of complications are related to the experience of the endoscopist
4. Even in experienced hands the procedure is not possible in 5–10% of cases
5. Can be performed via the afferent loop of a Polya gastrectomy
6. Previous sphincterotomy or sphincteroplasty may facilitate cannulation of the duodenal papilla
7. Close co-operation with an experienced radiologist is required for good results

Diagnostic ERCP
1. Pancreatic disease
   a. Chronic pancreatitis
      (i) Variations in the calibre of the pancreatic duct with beading
      (ii) Stricture with proximal dilatation of the pancreatic duct
      (iii) Defining the anatomy of the pancreatic duct is important in those patients being considered for surgical treatment
   b. Pancreatic carcinoma
      (i) Pancreatic carcinoma usually produces a localised stricture of the pancreatic duct and sometimes complete obstruction
      (ii) Dilatation of the pancreatic and/or common bile ducts due to distal obstruction is also commonly seen
   c. Pancreas divisum
      (i) Congenital abnormality occurring in up to 5% of the population
      (ii) May give rise to symptoms and predisposes to acute pancreatitis
2. Biliary disease
   a. Obstructive jaundice
      (i) In obstructive jaundice, oral or intra-venous cholangiography will not opacify the bile ducts
      (ii) ERCP is used in preference to percutaneous trans-hepatic cholangiography when there is no intra-hepatic duct dilatation
      (iii) It will show the site and extent of the obstructing lesion and often indicate its nature
   b. Intermittent cholestasis
   c. Post-cholecystectomy syndromes

Therapeutic ERCP
1. Endoscopic sphincterotomy
   a. Retained biliary calculi in common bile duct following cholecystectomy
   b. Primary common bile duct stones in elderly patients
   c. Papillary stenosis
   d. Papillary tumours
   e. Acute pancreatitis
2. Temporary drainage of an infected biliary tree
3. Insertion of permanent drainage prostheses
   a. Malignant strictures of extra-hepatic bile ducts
   b. Sclerosing cholangitis
4. Dilatation of biliary and pancreatic duct strictures

Complications

In addition to those of upper gastro-intestinal endoscopy, ERCP and the various therapeutic manoeuvres that can be performed have several specific complications. 10% of patients suffer significant complications but the overall mortality is less than 1%. In most series the mortality of endoscopic sphincterotomy for bile duct calculi is less than that of surgical exploration.

1. Ascending cholangitis
   a. Patients with biliary obstruction, especially if due to calculi, should receive prophylactic antibiotics to prevent this serious complication which is often rapidly followed by septicaemia
   b. If the obstruction is not successfully relieved urgent surgery is required
2. Acute pancreatitis
   a. Elevation of serum amylase is common but clinically significant acute pancreatitis complicates less than 1% of examinations
   b. It can be prevented by rigorous asepsis and avoidance of repeated injection of contrast or overfilling of the pancreatic duct
3. Haemorrhage
   a. Significant haemorrhage is the commonest complication of sphincterotomy occurring in 5–10% of patients
   b. Half of these patients require blood transfusion and one quarter need surgical exploration to arrest the bleeding
4. Retroperitoneal duodenal perforation

FURTHER READING

Leese T, Neoptolemos J P, Carr-Locke D L 1985 Successes, failures, early complications and their management following endoscopic sphincterotomy: results in 394 patients from a single centre. Br J Surg 72: 215–219

Leese T, Neoptolemos J P, Baker A R, Carr-Locke D L 1986 Management of acute cholangitis and the impact of endoscopic sphincterotomy. Br J Surg 73: 988–992

Cotton P B 1984 Endoscopic methods for relief of malignant obstructive jaundice. World J Surg 8: 854–861

Cotton P B, Bowden T A 1986 Gastrointestinal endoscopy and the surgeon. In Russell R C G (ed) Recent Advances in Surgery, Vol 12. Churchill Livingstone, Edinburgh pp 71–88

Cotton P B, Vallon A G 1982 Duodenoscopic sphincterotomy for removal of bile duct stones in patients with gall bladders. Surgery 91: 628–630

Goodall R J R 1985 Bleeding after endoscopic sphincterotomy. Ann R Coll Surg Eng 67: 87–88

Hamilton I 1986 Investigation of the pancreas: 2. ERCP, angiography and histology. Hosp Update 12: 399–403

Seifert E 1982 Endoscopy and biliary disease. In Blumgart L H (ed) The Biliary Tract. Clinical Surgery International No 5. Churchill Livingstone, Edinburgh pp 61–81
Thompson M H 1986 Influence of endoscopic papillotomy on the management of bile duct stones. Br J Surg 73: 779–781

ACUTE PANCREATITIS

Diagnostic criteria
1. Serum amylase > 1200 iu/l (1000 Somogyi units/l)
   a. In severe cases with extensive pancreatic destruction the serum amylase level may be normal
   b. Raised serum amylase levels may also be found in:
      (i) perforated peptic ulcer
      (ii) acute cholecystitis
      (iii) intestinal strangulation
      (iv) renal failure
      (v) ectopic pregnancy
      (vi) dissecting aortic aneurysm
      (vii) macroamylasaemia
2. Urinary amylase excretion > 3000 iu/l
3. Amylase:creatinine clearance ratio (ACCR) > 5%

With greater clinical awareness of the condition and more refined diagnostic techniques the proportion of patients with acute pancreatitis who remain undiagnosed until laparotomy is now less than 1%

Aetiological factors
1. Biliary tract disease
   a. Accounts for 40–50% of cases in United Kingdom
   b. The 'common channel' theory suggests that transient impaction of stones at the lower end of the common bile duct causes reflux of bile into the pancreatic duct
2. Alcohol
   a. Accounts for 25% of cases in this country
   b. Is a far more common cause of acute pancreatitis in the United States and France
   c. The mechanism by which alcohol produces acute pancreatitis remains unclear
3. Trauma
   a. Blunt abdominal injuries
   b. Penetrating abdominal trauma
4. Endoscopic retrograde cholangiopancreatography (ERCP)
   Acute pancreatitis complicates less than 1% of all ERCPs
5. Infections
   a. Viral, e.g. mumps virus, coxsackie B virus
   b. Bacterial, e.g. streptococcal septicaemia
6. Post-gastrectomy
   Obstruction to the afferent loop following Polya gastrectomy

7. Hypercalcaemia
8. Hyperlipidaemia
9. Drugs
  a. Corticosteroids
  b. Azathioprine
  c. Oral contraceptives
  d. Anti-coagulants
  e. Thiazide diuretics
10. Polyarteritis nodosa
11. Uraemia
12. Pancreas divisum

Management
1. Restore and maintain circulating blood volume
  a. Intra-venous crystalloids and colloids are given to maintain adequate arterial and central venous blood pressures
  b. Up to 5–10 litres of fluid may be required in the first 24 hours
  c. Albumin infusion may be required to maintain a satisfactory plasma colloid osmotic pressure
2. Monitor renal function
  a. Catheterise the patient and measure urine output hourly
  b. A urine output below 30 ml/h requires intra-venous mannitol providing the circulating blood volume has been restored
3. Suppress pancreatic exocrine secretions
  a. Naso-gastric aspiraton
  b. Anti-cholinergic drugs, e.g. atropine, propantheline are commonly used but are of no proven benefit
  c. Hormones such as glucagon and somatostatin similarly do not affect morbidity or mortality
  d. H_2-receptor antagonists, e.g. cimetidine, ranitidine
4. Analgesia
  a. Pethidine is used in preference to morphine which tends to stimulate the sphincter of Oddi
  b. Buprenorphine (Temgesic) is a useful alternative
5. Trasylol (Aprotonin)
  a. In an initial study this anti-protease drug which inhibits kallikrein and trypsin was shown to reduce the mortality of acute pancreatitis
  b. Two subsequent studies indicate that the drug is of no benefit
6. Antibiotics
  a. Routine use of prophylactic antibiotics does not prevent abscess formation
  b. Specific indications include ascending cholangitis and septicaemia

7. Peritoneal lavage
   a. Peritoneal lavage performed either at laparotomy or using a catheter inserted percutaneously is designed to remove proteolytic enzymes and toxins from the peritoneal cavity
   b. No improvement in either the morbidity or mortality of patients with severe acute pancreatitis is achieved when peritoneal lavage is used although the presence of protease inhibitors in the lavage fluid may prove to be of some benefit
8. Laparotomy
   a. Diagnostic laparotomy
      (i) Exploratory laparotomy has no therapeutic benefit
      (ii) It should not be performed unless the clinical diagnosis of acute pancreatitis is in doubt
   b. Biliary surgery
      (i) Cholecystectomy or cholecystostomy and choledochotomy with T-tube drainage may be necessary if the biliary tree is infected or obstructed
      (ii) In the presence of severe pancreatic inflammation most surgeons avoid sphincterotomy and sphincteroplasty
      (iii) Early biliary surgery, within 48–72 hours of the onset of an attack of acute gall stone pancreatitis, reduces the total length of hospitalisation and may reduce overall mortality
      (iv) It prevents the possibility of further attacks of pancreatitis whilst awaiting delayed surgery which is usually performed six weeks after the acute attack
      (v) Endoscopic papillotomy or sphincterotomy provides an alternative means of establishing adequate biliary drainage in acute pancreatitis
   c. Emergency pancreatic resection
      (i) Pancreatic sequestrectomy has been advocated in cases of very severe acute pancreatitis with extensive pancreatic necrosis
      (ii) Removal of necrotic pancreatic tissue, toxins and enzymes may prove helpful in some patients but it is often difficult to predict pre-operatively those in whom the procedure is likely to be beneficial
      (iii) Either subtotal or total pancreatectomy is performed depending on the findings at laparotomy
      (iv) Morbidity following emergency pancreatectomy for severe pancreatitis is high and the post-operative mortality is 20–40 per cent
9. Total parenteral nutrition (TPN)
   Intra-venous nutrition is indicated in those cases of severe pancreatitis which are slow to resolve or where surgical intervention is required

Complications
1. Acute oliguric renal failure
   a. Prevention by early and adequate restoration of the circulating blood volume is vitally important
   b. Established renal failure is treated by early peritoneal dialysis or haemodialysis
2. Cardio-respiratory failure
   a. Hypoxia may be severe and is often missed on clinical examination
   b. Repeated arterial blood gas analysis is essential in all cases of severe pancreatitis
   c. Treatment involves increasing the inspired pO_2 and if necessary intermittent positive pressure ventilation (IPPV)
   d. Inotropic agents, e.g. dopamine (Intropin), dobutamine (Dobutrex) may be required
3. Diabetes mellitus
   a. May be precipitated by infusion of hypertonic glucose solutions
   b. Managed with a continuous low-dose insulin infusion
4. Hypocalcaemia
   a. Serum calcium level is measured at frequent intervals especially if glucagon therapy is used
   b. Intra-venous calcium gluconate may be required
5. Pancreatic pseudocyst
   a. Peak incidence is 2–3 weeks after the start of an acute attack
   b. Seen in 10–20% of cases due to alcohol but less tha 5% of cases of gallstone pancreatitis
   c. Up to 50% will resolve spontaneously within 2 months
   d. Often associated with a persistently raised serum amylase level
   e. Diagnosis is confirmed by ultrasound examination
   f. Complications, which include rupture, haemorrhage and abscess formation, are more common in those patients suffering from gallstone pancreatitis and are associated with a 10% mortality
   g. When matured, pseudocysts can be drained surgically by cysto-gastrostomy or cysto-jejunostomy using a Roux loop
   h. Percutaneous drainage using a fine needle inserted under ultrasound or computed tomographic control is as effective as surgical drainage and can be performed at an earlier stage with less morbidity and mortality. Repeated aspirations may be necessary before the pseudocyst resolves completely
6. Pancreatic abscess
   a. A most serious complication associated with a mortality of over 50%
   b. Occurs in less than 5% of cases of acute pancreatitis occurring more commonly in cases of severe pancreatitis

   c. Presents with a swinging pyrexia and tachycardia along with a tender epigastric mass usually in the third or fourth week after the start of an acute attack

   d. Abscess may be multi-loculated and very extensive extending within the retroperitoneal tissues and having subphrenic, perinephric and pelvic components

   e. Diagnosis is confirmed by ultrasound or computed tomography

   f. Treatment comprises removal of all necrotic pancreatic tissue and external surgical drainage combined with intensive antibiotic therapy

   g. External drainage does not predispose to formation of a pancreatic fistula

7. Duodenal ileus

   a. Prolonged ileus suggests continuing pancreatic inflammation or abscess formation

   b. Naso-gastric aspiration and continued total parenteral nutrition are required

   c. A gastro-enterostomy or feeding jejunostomy may be indicated

8. Disseminated intra-vascular coagulation (DIC)

9. Gastro-intestinal haemorrhage

   a. Usually a terminal event

   b. Often associated with extensive pancreatic necrosis and abscess formation

10. Colonic and duodenal necrosis

Mortality

Mortality in acute pancreatitis is usually due to one or more of the following complications:

1. Irreversible shock
2. Acute oliguric renal failure
3. Cardio-respiratory failure
4. Retro-peritoneal abscess formation
5. Gastro-intestinal haemorrhage

The mortality rate is increased in elderly patients and is directly related to the severity of pancreatic inflammation:

Type of pancreatitis	Mortality rate (%)
Mild oedematous (interstitial)	1–2
Haemorrhagic	10–20
Necrotising	20–25

Prognostic factors

The degree of elevation of the serum amylase level is not related to the severity of the pancreatic inflammation. The following have been identified as indicators of a poor prognosis:

1. Arterial PO_2 < 60 mm Hg (8 kPa)
2. WBC   > 15 × 10⁹/l
3. Blood urea   > 16 mmol/l despite adequate fluid replacement
4. Blood glucose   > 10 mmol/l in the absence of previously diagnosed diabetes mellitus
5. Serum calcium   < 2.0 mmol/l
6. Serum albumin   < 32 g/l
7. Serum AST (GOT)   > 200 u/l
8. Serum LDH   > 600 iu/l

The presence of three or more of these factors within 48 hours of admission to hospital indicates severe acute pancreatitis. The greater the number of poor prognostic factors the higher is the risk of developing complications and the worse the patient's prognosis.

FURTHER READING

Aldridge M C, Ornstein M, Glazer G, Dudley H A F 1985 Pancreatic resection for severe acute pancreatitis. Br J Surg 72: 796–800

Baker R J, Duarte B 1986 The current status of recognition and treatment of severe necrotising pancreatitis. In: Nyhus L M (ed) Surgery Annual Vol 18. Appleton-Century-Crofts, Norwalk, Connecticut. pp 129–144

Carter D C 1983 Biliary tract surgery in gall-stone pancreatitis. Hosp Update 9: 879–893

Colhoun E, Murphy J J, MacEarlean D P 1984, Percutaneous drainage of pancreatic pseudocysts. Br J Surg 71: 131–132

Cumming J G R, Hamilton I 1986 Acute pancreatitis. Hosp Update 12: 949–964

Holdsworth P J, Meyer A D, Wilson D H, Flowers M W, McMahon M J 1984 A simple screening test for acute pancreatitis. Br J Surg 71: 958–959

Imrie C W 1985 Peritoneal lavage in severe acute pancreatitis. Br J Surg 72: 677

Imrie C W 1987 The role of surgery in pancreatitis. In: Taylor I (ed) Progress in Surgery Vol 2. Churchill Livingstone, Edinburgh pp 95–124

Imrie C W, Shearer M G 1986 Diagnosis and management of severe acute pancreatitis. In: Russell R C G (ed) Churchill Livingstone, Edinburgh pp 143–154

Kaushik S P, Vohra R, Verma G R, Kaushik S, Sabhrawal A 1984 Pancreatic abscesses: a review of seventeen cases. Br J Surg 71: 141–143

Nordback I H, Auvinen O A 1985 Long-term results after pancreas resection for acute necrotizing pancreatitis. Br J Surg 72: 687–689

Stone H H 1984 Immediate transduodenal sphincteroplasty for acute biliary pancreatitis. Dig Surg 1: 10–13

Wolfson P W 1980 Surgical management of inflammatory disorders of the pancreas. Surg Gynecol Obstet 151: 689–698

CHRONIC PANCREATITIS

Chronic pancreatitis is a continuing inflammatory process within the pancreas characterised by irreversible structural changes and causing pain and/or permanent loss of exocrine or endocrine function.

Aetiological factors
1. Excessive alcohol consumption accounts for more than 85% of all cases
2. Hypercalcaemia
3. Hyperlipidaemia
4. Protein-calorie malnutrition
5. Cystic fibrosis
6. Obstruction of pancreatic duct
   a. Congenital abnormalities such as malformation of the pancreatic duct, annular pancreas or pancreas divisum
   b. Tumours of the pancreas, ampulla or duodenum

Investigations
1. Plain abdominal radiography shows pancreatic calcification especially in cases of alcoholic pancreatitis
2. Pancreatic endocrine function is easily assessed using an oral glucose tolerance test
3. Assessment of pancreatic exocrine function
   a. Lundh test meal
   b. Secretin–cholecystokinin test
   c. 3-day faecal fat excretion
   d. Faecal enzyme measurements
4. Ultrasonography
   a. Ultrasound examination is abnormal in only half of all patients with chronic pancreatitis; this is often the result of technical difficulties preventing a satisfactory examination of the entire gland
   b. An enlarged echogenic pancreas is often seen
   c. A dilated pancreatic duct may also be visualised
5. Endoscopic retrograde cholangio-pancreatography (ERCP) Refer to Pages 31–32
   a. ERCP is abnormal in 85% of cases
   b. Side branches of the main pancreatic duct are shortened and often dilated whilst showing marked irregularities
   c. The main pancreatic duct is often severely deformed and irregular and may contain multiple strictures giving a 'chain of lakes' pattern
   d. Calculi within the pancreatic duct appear as filling defects
6. Computed tomography (CT)
   a. Pancreatic calcification is detected more readily than by plain radiography
   b. An enlarged pancreas and dilated pancreatic duct are common findings

Management
1. Identify and eliminate any predisposing causes; complete avoidance of alcohol is essential
2. Control of pain
   a. Simple oral analgesics may prove beneficial especially when combined with anti-cholinergic drugs
   b. Opiates may be required in some patients but there is a real risk of dependence
   c. Trans-cutaneous electrical nerve stimulation (TENS)
   d. Per-cutaneous or per-operative coeliac plexus block
   e. Splanchnicectomy
3. Maintain adequate nutritional status
4. Control diabetes mellitus if present
5. Oral pancreatic enzyme supplementation
   a. Examples include Pancrex V and Pancrease
   b. As they are destroyed by gastric acid their efficacy can be improved by simultaneous administration of antacids or H_2-receptor antagonists
6. Surgical drainage procedures
   a. These are designed to relieve pain due to ductal hypertension and a dilated pancreatic duct system whilst preserving the maximum amount of functioning pancreatic tissue
   b. Per-operative pancreatography may be required if adequate visualisation of the dilated duct system has not been achieved by pre-operative ERCP
   c. Trans-duodenal sphincterotomy or sphincteroplasty is indicated in those patients with ductal disease localised to the head of the pancreas and characterised by a short stricture adjacent to the duodenal papilla
   d. Distal pancreatectomy and lateral pancreatico-jejunostomy (Roux-en-Y) aims to achieve retrograde drainage of pancreatic juice in those patients with single strictures of the proximal pancreatic duct
   e. In an alternative pancreatico-jejunostomy the end of a Roux loop is anastomosed to the side of the pancreatic duct at the point of its maximum dilatation
   f. Longitudinal or side-to-side pancreatico-jejunostomy is required if the main pancreatic duct contains multiple strictures throughout its length
   g. Any associated pancreatic cysts should also be drained
7. Pancreatic resection
   a. Resection of pancreatic tissue aims to eliminate the disease process and so provide symptomatic relief of pain
   b. Further loss of functioning pancreatic tissue exaggerates the symptoms of pancreatic insufficiency
   c. Patients with disease predominantly confined to the body and tail of the pancreas may be suitable for distal pancreatectomy

   d. Major pancreatic resections are accompanied by a high
      post-operative morbidity and mortality and are therefore
      reserved for patients where previous operative treatment
      has failed or where the pancreatic duct is not dilated
   e. Pancreatico-duodenectomy normally involves resection of
      the head of the pancreas, duodenum and distal part of the
      stomach but in some cases it may be possible to preserve
      the pylorus and proximal duodenum
   f. Subtotal (distal) pancreatectomy which removes up to 95%
      of the gland leaving a cuff of pancreas along the medial
      aspect of the duodenum has a lower operative mortality
      than pancreatico-duodenectomy and produces similar
      symptomatic improvement

FURTHER READING

Cooper M J, Williamson R C N 1984 Drainage operations in chronic
   pancreatitis. Br J Surg 71: 761–766
Hamilton I 1986 Investigation of the pancreas: 1. Noninvasive techniques.
   Hosp Update 12: 299–308
Hamilton I 1986 Investigation of the pancreas: 2. ERCP, angiography, and
   histology. Hosp Update 12: 399–403
Hamilton I, Wormsley K G 1986 Chronic pancreatitis. Hosp Update
   12: 603–613
Imrie C W 1987 The role of surgery in pancreatitis. In: Taylor I (ed) Progress
   in Surgery Vol 2. Churchill Livingstone, Edinburgh pp 99–124
Wolfson P 1980 Surgical management of inflammatory disorders of the
   pancreas. Surg Gyn Obstet 151: 689–698

PANCREATIC CARCINOMA

Introduction

1. Carcinoma of the pancreas is a relatively common neoplasm
   with an incidence that is continuing to increase and a
   prognosis that is usually extremely poor
2. Median survival time irrespective of treatment is 2–4 months
   after the diagnosis has been made
3. 1-year survival is less than 10% and only 2% of patients survive
   5 years
4. Many patients are not suitable for surgical treatment at the
   time of presentation
5. Of those undergoing surgery 90% have regional lymph node
   metastases and 80% have hepatic metastases

Pre-operative diagnosis

70–85% of all cases of carcinoma arise in the head, neck or
uncinate process of the pancreas. Jaundice is therefore a common
presenting symptom. Even in those patients presenting with

obstructive jaundice an accurate pre-operative diagnosis is not always possible. Many investigations are available but only the first three are of routine clinical use.

1. Ultrasonography
   a. Tumours with a diameter of 2 cm or more are detectable by ultrasonography
   b. The technique is operator-dependent and in up to 25% of cases complete examination of the pancreas is prevented by overlying intestinal gas
   c. Fine needle percutaneous aspiration biopsy of a pancreatic mass is a safe and reliable technique which may be performed under ultrasound control
2. Computed tomography
   a. CT is generally more accurate than ultrasonography and gives more detailed information
   b. CT is usually a better imaging modality than ultrasonography for visualisation of the body and tail of the pancreas
   c. Like ultrasound it can also be used to guide fine needle percutaneous aspiration biopsy
   d. Features on CT which suggest that a pancreatic tumour is not resectable include hepatic or lymph node metastases, ascites and invasion of the superior mesenteric vessels, portal vein, inferior vena cava or aorta
3. Endoscopic retrograde cholangio-pancreatography (ERCP)
   a. Tumours invading the duodenum may be biopsied under direct vision
   b. Endoscopic transduodenal fine needle aspiration biopsy of the pancreas may yield positive evidence of a tumour in the pancreatic head
   c. Typical radiological features of pancreatic carcinomas include a localised stricture of the main pancreatic and common bile ducts with proximal dilatation; in some cases there is complete pancreatic duct occlusion
   d. Cytological examination of pure pancreatic juice aspirated from the main pancreatic duct further increases the diagnostic accuracy of ERCP
   e. In cases with obstructive jaundice ERCP may also be therapeutic allowing biliary drainage by insertion of either an endoprosthesis or a naso-biliary tube
4. Pancreatic function tests
   a. Pancreatic exocrine deficiency is present in 50% of cases of pancreatic carcinoma
   b. Available tests such as the Lundh test meal and the secretin–pancreozymin test fail to accurately differentiate between pancreatic carcinoma and chronic pancreatitis and are therefore no longer used routinely

5. Barium meal
   a. Tumours in the head of the pancreas may distort the duodenal loop
   b. The classical 'reversed three' sign is seen infrequently and barium meal examination now has little role in diagnosing pancreatic carcinoma
6. Radionuclide scintigraphy
   a. Pancreatic isotope scanning using ^{75}Se-selenomethionine is associated with a large number of false positive and false negative results
   b. It is therefore no longer used in the diagnosis of pancreatic carcinoma
7. Tumour markers
   a. Several tumour markers including carcino-embryonic antigen (CEA), pancreas cancer-associated antigen (PCCA) and pancreatic oncofetal antigen (POA) have been identified and may be associated with pancreatic carcinoma
   b. Each marker is not sufficiently specific or sensitive to be used to diagnose pancreatic carcinoma and as yet no reliable serological screening test is available
8. Laparoscopy
   a. Target biopsy of pancreatic lesions is readily performed
   b. Detection of intra-abdominal metastatic disease obviates unnecessary laparotomy
9. Angiography
   a. Either selective or superselective cannulation techniques are required to achieve satisfactory resolution
   b. When used as an initial diagnostic study the yield is relatively low
   c. Evidence of nonresectability may be obtained from angiography in cases where CT is not available

Per-operative diagnosis
At laparotomy, biopsy of pancreatic lesions is frequently avoided because of the dangers of acute pancreatitis and possible development of a pancreatic fistula. In addition the clinical diagnosis of pancreatic carcinoma is rarely incorrect in a jaundiced patient with a localised mass in the head of the pancreas and a dilated common bile duct which is thin walled and shows no signs of inflammation. In the occasional long-term survivor after palliative bypass surgery a diagnosis of pancreatic carcinoma may have been mistaken for chronic pancreatitis or a gall stone impacted at the lower end of the common bile duct.

Overall the complication rate of pancreatic biopsy is less than 10% and histological confirmation of a clinical diagnosis should always be sought. Various per-operative biopsy techniques are available.

1. Open wedge biopsy
   a. Suitable for abnormal pancreatic tissue which is easily accessible
   b. Complications following this method are rare
2. Thick needle (core) biopsy
   a. Indicated for deeply situated lesions
   b. Kocherisation of the duodenum allows a hand passed behind the pancreas to steady the gland whilst the Tru-Cut needle is passed into a lesion within the head of the pancreas
   c. Transduodenal biopsy is performed by passing the Tru-Cut needle through the lateral wall of the second part of the duodenum; following successful biopsy the puncture site in the duodenal wall is closed with a sero-muscular suture
   d. Biopsy material can be examined by frozen section
3. Fine needle aspiration biopsy
   a. Accurate puncture of the pancreatic lesion is again aided by mobilisation of the duodenum and pancreatic head
   b. Cytological examination of the aspirate gives a rapid diagnosis
4. Biopsy of suspected liver or peripancreatic lymph node metastases

Surgical treatment

(A) Curative treatment
Surgery is the only form of treatment that can potentially cure pancreatic carcinoma but usually less than 10% of patients present with lesions that are resectable. When curative surgical treatment is feasible long-term survival rates are low with fewer than 5% of patients surviving more than 5 years following curative surgery.
1. Subtotal pancreatectomy with duodenal resection (Whipple's procedure)
   a. Many surgeons reserve pancreatico-duodenectomy for periampullary duodenal carcinoma and adenocarcinoma of the distal common bile duct as these tumours have a more favourable prognosis than tumours of the pancreas, treating pancreatic lesions by palliative bypass procedures
   b. Pancreatico-duodenectomy involves en bloc removal of the duodenum, head and neck of the pancreas, antrum of the stomach, the gall bladder and common bile duct and the associated lymph nodes
   c. In general operative mortality rates are higher and the duration of hospital stay longer for patients undergoing resection than in those treated by palliative bypass
   d. Radical resection has an operative mortality of 10–20% but offers the only hope of cure in patients with pancreatic carcinoma and there are a few long term survivors

    e. Pancreatico-duodenectomy is probably the treatment of choice for a few carefully selected cases of carcinoma of the pancreatic head

2. Total pancreatectomy
    a. In addition to the structures removed during pancreatico-duodenectomy the remaining pancreas and spleen are removed in this operation
    b. Recurrence of tumour within the pancreas is also avoided and in general better lymph node clearance can be achieved
    c. Multicentric pancreatic tumours are treated effectively by total pancreatectomy
    d. Total pancreatectomy eliminates the risk of post-operative pancreatitis and avoids the possible complications associated with a pancreatico-jejunal anastomosis
    e. Complete exocrine and endocrine pancreatic failure always follows total pancreatectomy but exocrine pancreatic insufficiency and diabetes mellitus are common after the Whipple procedure
    f. No reduction in operative mortality or increased long term survival has been demonstrated in patients undergoing total pancreatectomy compared with those treated by Whipple's procedure

3. Radical extended or regional pancreatectomy
    a. In addition to removing the entire pancreas some or all of the three major vessels adjacent to the neck of the pancreas, portal vein, superior mesenteric artery and coeliac axis, are excised and reconstructed
    b. Although adoption of this procedure increases the operability of pancreatic tumours, post-operative mortality and morbidity are unacceptably high and there is no evidence of an overall benefit in survival

(B) Palliative surgical treatment
Indicated in patients with metastatic disease or inoperable tumours

1. Biliary–enteric bypass procedures
    a. Cholecysto-jejunostomy is the most commonly performed biliary drainage procedure
    b. Hepatodocho-jejunostomy is required in those cases where the cystic duct is occluded or likely to become invaded by the tumour

2. Gastro-enterostomy
    a. Duodenal obstruction is an unusual presenting feature of pancreatic carcinoma but is a well recognised complication of the later stages of the disease
    b. 15–35% of patients undergoing palliative biliary–enteric bypass will eventually require further surgery for duodenal obstruction: an additional 10–20% will die with symptomatic duodenal obstruction

    c. Operative mortality is not increased by routine concomitant gastro-enterostomy at the time of biliary-enteric bypass

    d. Routine prophylactic gastro-enterostomy will prevent the need for further surgery but has no effect on long-term survival

3. Intra-operative chemical splanchnicectomy

    a. Retroperitoneal extension of malignant disease to involve afferent nerve fibres around the coeliac axis produces a constant and often severe upper abdominal pain which radiates through to the back

    b. Injection of phenol or alcohol around the coeliac axis at the time of laparotomy relieves the pain in over 80% of patients, in most cases permanently: in contrast only 40% of patients undergoing biliary enteric bypass experienced relief of this distressing symptom

Radiotherapy

The main role of radiotherapy in pancreatic carcinoma is the palliation of pain. Radiotherapy is only indicated in the treatment of localised disease and in this rapidly debilitating disease a large proportion of patients are unsuitable for this form of treatment even at the time of diagnosis. The results of treatment are usually defined in terms of response rates rather than remission rates and even in the most encouraging reports increased survival is only a few weeks rather than several months.

1. External beam radiotherapy

    a. With low-energy (orthovoltage) machines it was impossible to deliver an adequate dose to the deeply situated pancreatic tumour without irradiating the intervening skin and other organs with unacceptably high doses

    b. Megavoltage radiotherapy has overcome these problems but to be effective accurate tumour localisation must be obtained; tumour volume may be defined at laparotomy by placing radio-opaque marker clips

    c. Accurate tumour localisation will minimise the risk of radiation damage to adjacent vital structures especially the spinal cord, stomach, small intestine, liver and kidneys

    d. Radiotherapy may have a role as an adjunct to the surgical treatment of pancreatic carcinoma

2. Interstitial radiotherapy

    a. Surgical implantation of radioactive sources into the tumour provides an alternative method of delivering a tumouricidal dose whilst limiting exposure to the adjacent normal tissues

    b. Implants of ^{125}I or ^{192}Au have been shown to palliate pain in some cases but significantly increased survival has not yet been documented

    c. Post-operative complications include pancreatitis, pancreatic fistula, duodenal obstruction and gastritis

3. Intra-operative radiotherapy
    a. Irradiation of surrounding normal tissues can also be reduced by this technique
    b. Sophisticated and expensive radiotherapy equipment is required to deliver high-energy electrons and is not generally available

Chemotherapy
1. Single agent chemotherapy
    a. The response rates of inoperable pancreatic carcinoma to single chemotherapeutic agents such as intra-venous 5-fluorouracil, nitrosoureas and mitomycin C are usually less than 20%
    b. Other single agents including methotrexate, methyl-CCNU and actinomycin D have no appreciable effect on pancreatic carcinoma
2. Combination chemotherapy
    a. Combination of agents such as 5-fluoruracil and methyl-CCNU or 5-fluorouracil and mitomycin C have yielded response rates up to 35%
    b. Response to combination chemotherapy is associated with a modest increase in length of survival
3. Adjuvant chemotherapy
    a. Chemotherapy may have an important role as an adjuvant to radiotherapy in control, of locally advanced pancreatic carcinoma
    b. Intra-venous 5-fluorouracil given on the first three days of a high dose course of radiotherapy has been shown to increase mean duration of survival by almost 100% compared with those patients receiving radiotherapy alone

Hormone therapy
Receptors for oestrogen, progesterone and androgen have all been identified in pancreatic carcinoma tissue and several preliminary studies have investigated the effects hormonal manipulation in the treatment of inoperable disease.
1. Anti-oestrogen therapy
    a. Two small studies have shown that tamoxifen (Novaldex) increases mean survival of patients with unresectable pancreatic carcinoma
    b. Further studies which contain larger numbers of patients are required to confirm this beneficial effect
2. Anti-androgen therapy
    a. LHRH analogues by lowering serum testosterone are effective in animal models of pancreatic carcinoma and may be of some value in the clinical situation
    b. A clinical trial of cyproterone acetate (Cyprostsat) has shown no effect on patient survival

FURTHER READING

Cuschieri A 1986 Carcinoma of the pancreas. Hosp Update 12: 453–458
Dobelbower R R, Milligan A J 1984 Treatment of pancreatic cancer by
    radiation therapy. World J Surg 8: 919–928
Gordis L, Gold E B 1984 Epidemiology of pancreatic cancer. World J Surg
    8: 808–821
Greenway B A 1987 Carcinoma of the exocrine pancreas: a sex hormone
    responsive tumour. Br J Surg 74: 441–442
Sarr M G, Cameron J L 1984 Surgical palliation of unresectable carcinoma
    of the pancreas. World J Surg 8: 906–918
Harvey J H, Schein P S 1984 Chemotherapy of pancreatic carcinoma. World
    J Surg 8: 935–939
Ihse I, Isaksson G 1984 Preoperative and operative diagnosis of pancreatic
    cancer. World J Surg 8: 846–853
Kummerle F, Ruckert K 1984 Surgical treatment of pancreatic cancer. World
    J Surg 8: 889–894
Longmire W P 1984 Cancer of the pancreas: palliative operation, Whipple
    procedure or total pancreatectomy. World J Surg 8: 872–879
Moosa A R, Scott M H, Lavelle-Jones M 1984 The place of total and
    extended total pancreatectomy in pancreatic cancer. World J Surg
    8: 895–899
Shipley W U, Tepper J E, Warshaw A L, Orlow E L 1984 Intraoperative
    radiation treatment for patients with pancreatic carcinoma. World J Surg
    8: 929–934

RETAINED BILIARY CALCULI

Prevention
Unsuspected biliary calculi are present in the common bile duct of
5–10% of patients undergoing elective cholecystectomy. Pre-
operative prediction of common bile duct stones is often unreliable
but they are readily detected by per-operative cholangiography
which should therefore always be performed routinely. This simple
investigation also allows recognition of any abnormal biliary
anatomy thus preventing accidental injury to the bile ducts.
Following surgical exploration of the common bile duct
choledochoscopy is performed to detect any residual calculi.

1. Per-operative cholangiography
   a. Normally performed by injecting contrast medium into the
      common bile duct via a cannula inserted into the cystic duct
   b. If cystic duct cholangiography is not technically possible
      contrast can be injected either into the gall bladder or
      directly into the common bile duct
   c. In addition to demonstrating the common hepatic and
      common bile ducts, both the right and left hepatic ducts
      with their main branches must be visualised
   d. Abnormal features suggesting the presence of stones in the
      hepatic or bile ducts include:
      (i) intraluminal filling defects
      (ii) dilated bile ducts

(iii) excessive retrograde filling of intra-hepatic bile ducts
(iv) lack of free flow of contrast into the duodenum
  e. Errors and misinterpretations include:
    (i) air bubbles introduced into the biliary system with the contrast
    (ii) superimposition of the opacified biliary tree on the vertebral column can be prevented by rotating the operating table 15° to the right
    (iii) misinterpretation of the normally narrowed terminal segment of the common bile duct
2. Per-operative biliary endoscopy (cholangioscopy or choledochoscopy)
  a. Not an alternative to per-operative cholangiography. (Choledochotomy should not be performed only to permit introduction of the choledochoscope.)
  b. Either a rigid or a flexible endoscope may be used; Kocherisation of the duodenum facilitates examination of the distal part of the common bile duct especially if a rigid choledochoscope is used
  c. Choledochoscopy is generally used to confirm that the biliary tree is free of calculi following conventional surgical exploration of the bile ducts. (Post-exploratory T-tube cholangiography is notoriously unreliable as it is difficult to exclude air bubbles.)
  d. Balloon catheters, Dormia baskets and biopsy forceps can be used to remove biliary calculi endoscopically

Treatment
Retained biliary calculi are found in 5–10% of all patients who have undergone exploration of the common bile duct and are usually discovered at routine T-tube cholangiography which is performed 7–10 days after surgery. Small calculi in the distal part of the common bile duct may pass spontaneously and are not seen on repeat cholangiography. Calculi which persist should be removed by one of the following techniques
1. Mechanical flushing with normal saline
  a. Suitable for small stones, generally those less than 5 mm in diameter, situated between the distal limb of the T-tube and the duodenum
  b. Infusion pressure should be carefully monitored and must not exceed 30 cm H_2O
  c. The procedure should be abandoned if the patient experiences pain
  d. Increased flow rates may be obtained by relaxation of the sphincter of Oddi using glucagon or ceruletide in those patients who have not undergone sphincterotomy
  e. Addition of heparin to the perfusate does not increase the success rate
  f. Overall success rates of 50–60% are usually reported

2. Contact dissolution with solvents
   a. 100 mM sodium cholate solution infused at 30 ml/h has been used to dissolve cholesterol stones situated on either side of the T-tube
   b. Serial T-tube cholangiograms are used to monitor progress of the treatment which may take up to 14 days
   c. Aqueous solutions of other bile salts such as sodium deoxycholate and sodium chenodeoxycholate have been used but all produce considerable diarrhoea
   d. Other agents with even greater solubility for cholesterol have recently been used for contact dissolution; examples include mono-octanoin, D-limonene and methyl-t-butyl-ether (MTBE)
   e. Dissolution of pigment stones requires use of chelating agents such as ethylenediaminetetra-acetic acid (EDTA) in addition to cholesterol solvents
3. Percutaneous extraction
   a. An interventional radiological technique performed under light sedation
   b. The T-tube must be left in situ for at least 6 weeks to allow its tract to mature
   c. Technique is simplified if the tract is wide and straight: a T-tube of at least size 14 FG should always be used and it is exteriorised through the lateral abdominal wall to prevent tortuosity of the tract and to minimise exposure of the radiologist's hands to ionising radiation
   d. The tract of a smaller tube may require dilatation prior o instrumentation
   e. Immediatley following removal of the T-tube a steerable Burhenne catheter is inserted along its tract and into the common bile duct
   f. A Dormia basket is passed along the catheter and is used to retrieve the stones
   g. Repeat cholangiography is used to confirm complete clearance of stones after which the catheter is removed and the tract closes spontaneously
   h. In expert hands the overall success rate is 95%
   i. Complications occur in about 5% of cases and include cholangitis, pancreatitis and leakage of bile from the sinus tract leading to bile collections and peritoneal contamination. (Fatal complications are very rare.)
   j. Passage of a choledochoscope along a matured T-tube tract has also been reported with removal of a retained calculus by a Dormia basket under direct vision
4. Endoscopic sphincterotomy
   a. A relatively safe technique which can be performed in the early post-operative period
   b. After endoscopic retrograde cholangiography (ERCP) is performed to identify the position, size and number of

retained stones a sphincterotome is introducd into the
ampulla of Vater and sphincterotomy performed
- c. The T-tube is then removed and the calculi are extracted
using a balloon catheter or Dormia basket
- d. Successful clearance of retained stones is confirmed by
repeat cholangiography and is usually achieved in 85–90%
of cases
- e. Complications which include haemorrhage, pancreatitis and
cholangitis occur in 5–10% of patients
5. Further surgical exploration
- a. Indication when non-operative methods are unavailable or
are either not feasible or prove unsuccessful
- b. Choledochotomy should be combined with adequate
drainage of the common bil duct either by sphincterotomy
and sphincteroplasty or choledocho-duodenostomy

The second group of patients with retained biliary calculi are those
who have not undergone choledochotomy at the time of
cholecystectomy. Symptoms occur either in the early post-
operative period or at a later date and are normally accompanied
by features of obstructive jaundice.

1. Endoscpic sphincterotomy
- a. Should always be considered as the first line treatment in
this group of patients especially the elderly and those of
high risk
- b. Can be performed immediately after diagnostic ERCP
2. Surgical exploration
- a. Further surgery is usually performed if endoscopic
sphincterotomy has failed or electively after ERCP in
younger patients especially those with large gall stones or a
grossly dilated common bile duct
- b. Supra-duodenal choledochotomy is combined with a biliary
enteric anastomosis to provide internal biliary drainage
- c. Choledocho-duodenostomy is the preferred method of
biliary drainage if the diameter of the common bile duct
exceeds 1.5 cm as it avoids the risk of acute pancreatitis
associated with transduodenal sphincterotomy and
sphincteroplasty
- d. Transduodenal sphincterotomy and sphincteroplasty are
performed if the common bile duct is less than 1.5 cm in
diameter or if a stone is impacted in the ampulla of Vater

FURTHER READING

Allison D J, Bowley N B 1982 Interventional radiology in biliary tract
disease. In: Blumgart L H (ed) Clinical Surgery International No 5 The
Biliary Tract. Churchill Livingstone, Edinburgh pp 82–98
Blumgart L H, Lygidakis N J 1982 The post-cholecystecomy patient. In:

Blumgart L H (ed) Clinical Surgery International No 5 The Biliary Tract. Churchill Livingstone, Edinburgh pp 143–156

Britton B J 1987 The management of stones in the common bile duct. In: Taylor I (ed) Progress in Surgery Vol 2. Churchill Livingstone, Edinburgh pp 86–98

Ashby B S 1985 Operative choledochoscopy in common bile duct surgery. Ann R Coll Surg Eng 67: 279–283

Johnson A G, Hosking S W 1987 Appraisal of the management of bile duct stones. Br J Surg 74: 555–560

Morgenstern L, Berci G 1982 Intraoperative diagnostic procedures. In: Blumgart L H (ed) Clinical Surgery International No 5 The Biliary Tract. Churchill Livingstone, Edinburgh pp 99–120

Neoptolemos J P, Hofmann A F, Moosa A R 1986 Chemical treatment of stones in the biliary tree. Br J Surg 73: 515–524

O'Doherty D P, Neoptolemos J P, Carr-Locke D L 1986 Endoscopic sphincterotomy for retained common bile duct stones in patients with T-tube in situ in the early postoperative period. Br J Surg 73: 454–456

Summerfield J A 1985 Endoscopic management of gall stones. Hosp Update 11: 693–703

SPLENECTOMY

Indications
1. Rupture of spleen
   a. Traumatic rupture
      (i) Accidental trauma
      (ii) Iatrogenic trauma
   b. Spontaneous rupture
      Trivial injury to a pathologically enlarged spleen, e.g. malaria, infectious mononucleosis
2. Primary hypersplenism
   Abnormal formed elements of the blood are removed by a normal spleen:
   a. Idiopathic thrombocytopenic purpura (ITP)
   b. Haemolytic anaemias
      (i) hereditary spherocytosis
      (ii) hereditary elliptocytosis
      (iii) auto-immune haemolytic anaemia
      (iv) β-thalassaemia major
      (v) sickle cell disease
      (vi) pyruvate kinase deficiency
3. Secondary hypersplenism
   Normal formed elements of the blood are removed inappropriately by an abnormal and usually enlarged spleen:
   a. Chronic lymphocytic leukaemia (CLL)
   b. Chronic granulocytic leukaemia (CGL)
   c. Malignant lymphoma
   d. Myelofibrosis
   e. Hairy cell leukaemia (leukaemic reticuloendotheliosis)
   f. Felty's syndrome

    g. Banti's Syndrome

    h. Lipid storage diseases

       In giant splenomegaly splenectomy may be required to relieve the symptoms attributable to the presence of a large intra-abdominal mass.

4. Splenectomy as part of staging laparotomy for Hodgkin's disease and other lymphomas
5. Splenectomy as part of other surgical procedures
   a. Radical surgery for gastric and oesophageal carcinomas
   b. Distal pancreatectomy
   c. Portal decompression by conventional spleno-renal shunt
6. Splenic abscesses, cysts and tumours
   a. Pyogenic abscess
   b. Hydatid cyst
   c. Congenital cyst
   d. Degenerative cyst
   e. Splenic haemangioma
7. Immunosuppression
   Splenectomy may enhance survival of cadaveric renal allografts
8. Diagnostic splenectomy
   a. Undiagnosed splenomegaly
   b. Pyrexia of unknown origin (PUO)
     With improved investigative techniques, especially imaging by computed tomography, diagnostic splenectomy is rarely required

Surgical technique

1. Upper midline incision is used in emergency surgery, for splenectomy as part of staging laparotomy, in cases of massive splenomegaly and if cholecystectomy is to be performed at the same time. A left subcostal incision can be used for elective removal of small spleens
2. Lieno-renal ligament is divided allowing the spleen to be mobilised into the wound
3. Short gastric vessels are divided
4. Splenic pedicle is dissected and the main splenic vessels ligated and divided
5. Drainage of the splenic bed is indicated if there is inadequate haemostasis, damage to the tail of the pancreas, or contamination of the splenic bed by gastro-intestinal contents
6. In cases of primary hypersplenism a careful search for splenunculi must be made

Complications

The incidence and nature of complications are closely related to the indication for splenectomy and the presence of other associated diseases. The high incidence of complications following splenectomy for traumatic rupture is due to the associated thoracic and other intra-abdominal injuries. Patients with hypersplenism are often poor operative risks because of anaemia, thrombocytopenia, prolonged steroid therapy or advanced malignant disease.

1. Haemorrhage
    a. Excessive operative blood loss may be due to:
        (i) Vascular adhesions between the spleen and the diaphragm
        (ii) Retroperitoneal porta-systemic anastomoses in cases of portal hypertension
        (iii) Difficult exposure of the splenic vessels, especially likely in very large spleens
    b. Post-operative haemorrhage is due to:
        (i) Poor surgical technique
        (ii) Coagulation defects, especially thrombocytopenia
2. Pulmonary atelectasis
    a. Left lower lobe pulmonary collapse often with consolidation is usually associated with a small ipsilateral pleural effusion
    b. Irritation of the left hemidiaphragm impairs its movement
    c. Hypoventilation due to rib fractures should be prevented in traumatic cases by aggressive chest physiotherapy
3. Subphrenic abscess
    a. Occurs in less than 1% of all elective splenectomies
    b. Routine drainage of the splenic bed does not reduce its incidence
4. Post-splenectomy fever
    a. Post-operative pyrexia is most likely to represent a chest or wound infection or the presence of a subphrenic abscess
    b. A minority of patients suffer an otherwise unexplained pyrexia which lasts up to three weeks: it may be caused by leucocyte agglutinating antibodies normally removed by the spleen
5. Thrombocytosis
    a. The platelet count is usually elevated in the first two weeks after splenectomy
    b. In some patients thre is an exaggerated rise sometimes reaching levels of $2,000 \times 10^9/l$
    c. These patients are at increased risk of developing deep vein thrombosis, pulmonary embolism and less commonly mesenteric vein thrombosis
    d. Patients with a platelet count greater than $750 \times 10^9/l$ should receive either aspirin 300 mg daily or dipyridamole (Persantin) 100 mg 6-hourly until the count falls below this level
6. Overwhelming post-splenectomy sepsis
    a. Although splenectomised children are at the highest risk, this serious complication is now well recognised in patients undergoing splenectomy in adult life

    b. Often an abrupt onset and running a fulminant course despite antibiotic treatment

    c. The source of infection is rarely identified but the causative organism is a pneumococcus in 50% of cases

    d. Other bacteria known to be associated with overwhelming infection in splenectomised patients include *Neisseria meningitidis, Escherichia coli* and *Haemophilus influenzae*

    e. May be fatal within 24–48 hours of onset, death being associated with disseminated intra-vascular coagulation (DIC) and bilateral adrenal haemorrhage

    f. Greatest risk is in the first two years following splenectomy but splenectomised patients remain at risk indefinitely

    g. Increased susceptibility to infection is due to decreased tuftsin production, impaired IgM antibody synthesis and a reduced ability to clear particulate matter from the blood stream

    h. Prophylaxis with either penicillin V or a polyvalent pneumococcal vaccine is recommended; vaccines against other pathogens such as Haemophilus influenzae and Neisseria meningitidis are also available

7. Pancreatic fistula

    a. May occur if the tail of the pancreas is damaged during exposure and ligation of the splenic vessels at the hilum

    b. Adequate drainage is normally followed by spontaneous closure

8. Gastric fistula

    a. An extremely rare complication

    b. May occur if part of the greater curvature of the stomach is devascularised by the ligatures securing the short gastric vessels

FURTHER READING

Mitchell A, Morris P J 1983 Surgery of the spleen. Clinics in Haematology 12: 565–589

Cooper M J, Williamson R C N 1984 Splenectomy: indications hazards and alternatives. Br J Surg 71: 173–180

Schwartz S I 1981 Splenectomy for hematologic disease. Surg Clin N Am 61: 117–125

PORTAL HYPERTENSION

The hepatic portal vein is formed by the union of the superior mesenteric and splenic veins and drains blood from most of the gastro-intestinal tract, spleen, pancreas and gall bladder. The portal venous pressure is normally about 7 mm Hg and blood flows through the portal vein at a rate of 1000–1200 ml/minute. Any obstruction to the flow of portal venous blood results in portal hypertension.

Classification

Pre-sinusoidal portal hypertension

1. Pre-hepatic obstruction
   a. portal vein thrombosis
      (i) congenital malformation
      (ii) neonatal umbilical sepsis
      (iii) umbilical vein catheterisation
      (iv) tumour invasion
      (v) hypercoagulable states
      (vi) trauma
      (vii) intra-abdominal sepsis
      (viii) thrombosed porto-caval shunt
   b. Splenic vein thrombosis
      (i) trauma
      (ii) lymphoma
      (iii) splenectomy
2. Intra-hepatic obstruction
   a. Congenital hepatic fibrosis
   b. Schistosomiasis
   c. Primary biliary cirrhosis
   d. Sarcoidosis
   e. Myelo-proliferative diseases
   f. Toxins, e.g. vinyl chloride, copper, arsenic

Intra-hepatic portal hypertension

1. Cirrhosis
2. Chronic active hepatitis

Post-hepatic (post-sinusoidal) portal hypertension

1. Veno-occlusive disease
2. Hepatic vein thrombosis (Budd–Chiari syndrome)
   a. spontaneous
   b. tumour invasion
   c. oral contraceptives
   d. hypercoagulable states
3. Congestive cardiac failure
4. Constrictive pericarditis

Clinical features

1. Features of hepato-cellular failure (absent in cases of portal venous occlusion)
   a. Jaundice
   b. Hyperkinetic circulation
   c. Hepatic encephalopathy
2. Splenomegaly
   a. The diagnosis of portal hypertension is questionable in the absence of splenomegaly

b. The actual size of an enlarged spleen is not necessarily directly related to the degree of portal hypertension
3. Hepatomegaly
   a. Liver size correlates poorly with the degree of portal hypertension
   b. Although hepatomegaly may accompany portal hypertension marked increases in portal venous pressure are usually associated with a small, shrunken and fibrotic liver
4. Ascites
5. Dilated superficial veins on anterior abdominal wall
   a. Blood flow in a caput Medusae is centrifugal
   b. A venous murmur may be audible

Prognostic criteria (Child's classification)

	Group A	Group B	Group C
Serum bilirubin	< 25 μmol/l	25–50 μmol/l	> 50 μmol/l
Serum albumin	> 35 g/l	30–35 g/l	<30 g/l
Ascites	None	Easily controlled	Poorly controlled
Encephalopathy	None	Mild or moderate	Advanced
Nutrition	Excellent	Good	Poor
Operative risk	Good	Moderate	Poor

1. Prognosis following acute variceal haemorrhage and after both emergency and elective surgery is closely related to hepatic function
2. Patients with pre-hepatic portal hypertension where liver function is usually well preserved have low operative mortality and morbidity
3. In patients with alcoholic cirrhosis abstention from alcohol and appropriate medical treatment can significantly improve hepatic function and therefore prognostic criteria

Emergency management of variceal haemorrhage
1. Resuscitation of hypovolaemic patient
   a. Intra-venous infusion of colloids
   b. Blood transfusion using fresh blood if available
2. Correction of coagulation defects
   a. Fresh frozen plasma
   b. Intra-venous vitamin K
   c. Platelet concentrates

3. Prevention of hepatic encephalopathy
   a. Magnesium sulphate
   b. Lactulose
   c. Enteral antibiotics, e.g. neomycin, metronidazole
   d. Intra-venous infusion of dextrose solutions is used to prevent hypogylcaemia
4. Endoscopic diagnosis
   a. Up to 25% of patients with oesophageal or gastric varices may bleed from other sites especially duodenal ulcers and superficial gastric erosions
   b. Urgent and accurate endoscopic assessment is therefore important in all cases
   c. Varices are only accepted as the source of haemorrhage if they are actively bleeding or if blood clot is adherent to the overlying oesophageal mucosa
5. Vasopressin (Pitressin)
   a. Reduces portal venous pressure by constricting splanchnic arterioles
   b. Causes contraction of oesophageal musculature with reduced variceal blood flow
   c. Decreases hepatic and coronary arterial blood flow
   d. May be given as an intra-venous bolus (20 units in 100 ml 5% dextrose over 2–20 minutes) or by continuous intra-venous infusion (0.4 units/minute) which may be more effective
   e. Intra-arterial injection offers no advantage
   f. Haemorrhage is controlled in 50% of patients but recurrence is very common
   g. Complications include ischaemic colitis and emphysematous gastritis
   h. Triglycyl lysine vasopressin (Glypressin) given by intermittent bolus injection (2 mg 6-hourly) is longer acting and has fewer side effects
6. Gastro-oesophageal balloon tamponade
   a. Linton–Nachlas tube which has a large gastric but no oesophageal balloon is useful for gastric varices
   b. Sengstaken–Blakemore tube and its various modifications which have both gastric and oesophageal balloons are useful for oesphageal varices
   c. Successful control of haemorrhage can be obtained in over 80% of cases but rebleeding occurs in half and overall mortality is 50%
   d. Tamponade is therefore usually used only as a temporary measure prior to more definitive therapy
   e. Tubes must not be inflated for more than 24 hours
   f. Following deflation the tube is left in situ and the balloon reflated if haemorrhage recurs
   g. Complications include aspiration pneumonia, oesophageal ulceration and rupture of the oesophagus

7. Endoscopic injection sclerotherapy
   a. Over the past ten years this has become the initial treatment of choice for acute variceal haemorrhage
   b. It effectively controls haemorrhage in up to 95% of cases
   c. A rigid oesophagoscope or flexible fibre-optic endoscope with or without a sheath is used to inject sodium tetradecyl sulphate (STD), ethanolamine oleate or sodium morrhuate into (intra-variceal injection) or around the varices (para-variceal injection)
   d. Temporary osophageal tamponade may be required as an adjunctive measure
   e. Compared with standard medical treatment injection sclerotherapy reduces rebleeding and mortality rates by over 50%
   f. Complications include oesophageal perforation, ulceration and stricture formation
8. Percutaneous trans-hepatic obliteration of varices
   a. Requires considerable technical expertise
   b. Can be performed in poor risk patients
   c. Not feasible if portal vein is occluded
   d. Catheter is passed under local anaesthetic through the liver and via the portal vein into the left and short gastric veins
   e. Following selective catheterisation, vessels supplying the varices are obliterated by injection of thrombin, gelatine foam, isobutylcyanoacrylate or lyophilised dura mater
   f. Control of bleeding is obtained in 75% of patients but recurrence occurs in half
   g. Complications include intra-peritoneal haemorrhage, biliary peritonitis, pulmonary emboli and pleural effusion
9. Ligation of varices
   a. The transthoracic transoesophageal (Boerema–Crile operation) involves suturing the varices having gained access via a longitudinal oesophagomyotomy
   b. Milnes–Walker modification involves complete mucosal transection to aid variceal ligation
   c. Despite various modifications these procedures when used in the emergency situation are associated with operative mortality rates of 40–50%
10. Oesophageal transection and anastomosis
    a. Initially performed using conventional suturing techniques or the Boerema button but now usually peformed with the American EEA stapling device or the Russian SPTU gun which greatly simplify the procedure
    b. The abdominal oesophagus is mobilised at laparotomy and the vagal trunks preserved to avoid the need for a separate gastric drainage procedure
    c. Stapling instrument is introduced through an anterior gastrotomy and advanced into the distal oesophagus

d. Transection is performed at the oesophago-gastric junction or immediately above it
e. Encephalopathy is not precipitated but the operative mortality for emergency surgery is approximately 30%

11. Devascularisation procedures
a. Various devascularisation procedures are available and are normally combined with either an oesophageal or gastric transection procedure
b. Subcardiac porto-azygos disconnection (Tanner operation) involves proximal gastric transection and reanastomosis in addition to ligation of the left gastric artery and vein and the short gastric vessels
c. Sugiura procedure is a more extensive devascularisation procedure, the oesophagus being devascularised via a trans-thoracic approach to the level of the inferior pulmonary vein, transected and resutured. Through a separate laparotomy incision splenectomy is performed followed by devascularisation of the proximal stomach, selective vagotomy and pyloroplasty

12. Emergency porta-systemic shunt surgery
a. Rarely performed due to the excessively high operative mortality
b. Emergency end-to-side porta-caval anastomosis has a 50% mortality rate: surviving patients have a minimal risk of rebleeding but severe porto-systemic encephalopathy occurs in many cases
c. Placing an interposition Dacron ('jump') graft between the superior mesenteric vein and the inferior vena cava (mesenterico-caval shunt) has a 30–40% operative mortality rate

Elective treatment of portal hypertension

Medical
1. β-adrenergic receptor blockers such as propanolol will reduce cardiac output and splanchnic blood flow
2. Propanolol has been shown to reduce portal venous pressure
3. French studies have claimed that porpanolol reduces the rate of future bleeding from oesophageal varices and improves long-term survival in patients with portal hypertension
4. Further trials involving larger numbers of patients are required before the exact role of beta-blockers in portal hypertension is determined

Injection sclerotherapy
1. Repeated sclerotherapy at 1–4 weekly intervals until all the varices disappear reduces the indicence of further haemorrhage

2. Frequently repeated injections are liable to cause mucosal ulceration
3. One trial has shown that repeated injection sclerotherapy significantly improves long-term survival of patients with varices

Porta-systemic decompression
1. Shunt surgery offers maximal protection against further variceal bleeding provided the porta-systemic fistula remains patent
2. In cases of hepatic disease, prevention of further variceal haemorrhage is usually achieved only at the expense of an increased risk of hepatic encephalopathy
3. Though often performed in the USA porta-systemic shunting procedures are rarely carried out in the UK
4. Young patients with pre-hepatic portal hypertension and normal liver function may be considered for elective shunt surgery if other methods of treatment had failed to prevent recurrent variceal haemorrhage
5. The operative mortality of elective porta-systemic decompression remains high, about 20% in most series, and surgery is contraindicated in the following situations:
   a. acute variceal haemorrhage
   b. porta-systemic encephalopathy
   c. schistosomiasis
   d. diabetes mellitues
   e. patients over 50 years
   f. Child's grade C
6. Porta-caval shunt
   a. Patent portal vein must be demonstrated pre-operatively by portal venography or ultra-sound scan
   b. An end-to-side shunt is normally created; a side-to-side shunt is technically more difficult to perform and offers no definite advantage
   c. Operative mortality rate is 10–20%
   d. Further variceal haemorrhage occurs in less than 5% of patients
   e. 25–50% of surviving patients will develop porta-systemic encephalopathy
   f. The combined results of three USA controlled trials showed that porta-caval shunting increases long-term survival to a small extent
7. Interposition mesenterico-caval shunt (H-graft)
   a. May be required if the portal vein or a previous porta-caval shunt has thrombosed
   b. Wide bore prosthetic material or autogenous saphenous vein is inserted between the superior mesenteric vein and the inferior vena cava ('jump' graft)

   c. Continued hepatic portal venous flow preserves liver function and a low incidence of encephalopathy is seen

   d. High patency rates are usually achieved and therefore rebleeding is uncommon

8. Conventional lieno-renal shunt
   a. Splenic vein must be patent
   b. Incidence of rebleeding is higher than after porta-caval shunt and is probably related to 20% incidence of shunt thrombosis
   c. Operative mortality is similar to that of porta-caval shunting but the incidence of encephalopathy is reduced to approximately 10%

9. Selective (distal) lieno-renal shunt (Warren's operation)
   a. An attempt at selective decompression of gastro-oesphageal varices without disturbing mesenteric or portal venus flow
   b. Theoretically this should minimise the risk of porta-systemic encephalopathy and by maintaining hepatic blood flow not impair liver function
   c. Splenic vein must be patent
   d. Operative mortality and survival rates are similar to those of other shunt procedures but the incidence of encephalopathy is reduced to 10–15%

Oesophageal transection and anastomosis
   a. Can be used in patients who are considered unsuitable for elective shunt surgery
   b. Transection with a stapling instrument may be combined with devascularisation of the lower oesophagus and upper part of the stomach
   c. Coincidental splenectomy is performed if significant hypersplenism is present
   d. Post-operative complicatons include oesophageal stricture and anastomotic leakage
   e. Porta-systemic encephalopathy is not a significant complication
   f. Operative mortality for elective surgery is less than 10%

FURTHER READING

Spence R A J, Johnston G W 1986 Oesophageal varices: pathogenesis and management. In: Russell R C G (ed) Recent Advances in Surgery Vol 12. Churchill Livingstone, Edinburgh pp 105–123
Spence R A J, Anderson J R, Johnston G W 1985 Twenty-five years of injection sclerotherapy for bleeding varices. Br J Surg 72: 195–198
Johnston G W 1982 Six years' experience of oesophageal transection for oesophageal varices using a circular stapling gun. Gut 23: 770–773
Larson G M 1986 Injection sclerotherapy for oesophageal varices: an

update. In: Nyhus L M (ed) Surgery Annual 1986. Appleton-Century-Crofts, Norwalk, Connecticut pp 351–376

McLaren M I, Taylor I 1986 Advances in managing variceal bleeding in portal hypertension. In: Nyhus L M (ed) Surgery Annual 1986. Appleton-Century-Crofts, Norwalk, Connecticut pp 243–277

McLaren M I, Taylor I 1986 The management of portal hypertension and bleeding varices. In: Taylor I (ed) Progress in Surgery Vol 1 Churchill Livingstone, Edinburgh pp 67–84

Joffe S N 1984 Non-operative management of variceal bleeding. Br J Surg 71: 85–91

Sherlock S 1983 Management of bleeding oesophageal varices. Hosp Update 9: 1213–1218

Umeyama K, Yoshikawa K, Yamashita T, Todo T, Satake K 1983 Transabdominal oesophageal transection for oesophageal varices: experience in 101 patients. Br J Surg 70: 419–422

Colorectal surgery

COLONOSCOPY

Technique
1. Performed under intra-venous sedation and radiological control if required
2. Adequate mechanical bowel preparation is an essential pre-requisite for a satisfactory examination
3. The flexible fibre-optic colonoscope is normally introduced per rectum but it can be inserted via a terminal or loop colostomy or ileostomy
4. Expert endoscopists can visualise the entire colon in over 90% of cases

Indications for diagnostic colonoscopy
1. Investigation of patients with abnormal or equivocal barium enema examinations
   a. Colonoscopy can be used to confirm or exclude carcinoma in a segment of colon affected by diverticular disease
   b. Direct visualisation of the abnormal area is combined with mucosal biopsy
2. Investigation of symptomatic patients with normal barium enema examinations
   a. Endoscopy is able to localise the source of unexplained blood loss
   b. It is also used to investigate patients with unexplained abdominal pain or diarrhoea
3. Investigation of patients with proven large bowel carcinoma
   a. Colonoscopy is important in the search for synchronous lesions both adenomas and further carcinomas
   b. These may be present in up to 25% and 5% of patients respectively
4. Post-colonic resection surveillance
   a. Colonoscopy is used to search for adenomas, metachronous carcinomas or suture line recurrence in patients who have previously undergone colonic resection for adenocarcinoma

    b. Initial colonoscopy should be performed after a few months to inspect the suture line and exclude any lesions missed at the pre-operative assessment

    c. Optimal frequency of further examinations is not yet detemined

5. Post-polypectomy surveillance

    a. Colonoscopic surveillance is essential to search for further polyps in those patients who have previously undergone excision of adenomatous polyps and especially in cases showing malignant change

    b. The ideal frequency of further follow-up examinations is still not finally determined but should be related to the degree of risk e.g. 2-yearly for high-risk patients and 4-yearly for low-risk patients

6. Assessment of inflammatory bowel disease

    a. To estimate the extent of colonic involvement in ulcerative colitis

    b. To obtain regular multiple colonic biopsies from patients with total colitis so that prophylactic colectomy can be performed if dysplasia develops

    c. To biopsy all strictures in colitic patients

    d. To accurately assess colonic segments affected by Crohn's disease

Indications for therapeutic colonoscopy

1. Polypectomy

    a. Performed using a diathermy snare, this procedure has a relatively low morbidity and mortality

    b. It is therefore preferable to laparotomy, colotomy and surgical polypectomy in those patients with polyps inaccessible to the operating sigmoidoscope

2. Treatment of caecal and sigmoid volvulus
3. Deflation of colonic pseudo-obstruction
4. Removal of foreign bodies
5. 'Hot biopsy' of telangiectasia
6. Electro-coagulation of bleeding points
7. Dilatation of colonic strictures

Contraindications

1. Recent myocardial infarction
2. Acute intestinal obstruction
3. Peritonitis
4. Acute colitis or diverticulitis
5. Recent abdominal surgery

Complications

1. Perforation
   a. Perforation occurs in 0.2% of cases and requires urgent laparotomy
   b. The sigmoid colon is the site most frequently perforated
   c. Risk is increased in the presence of underlying disease such as radiation colitis, inflammatory bowel disease of diverticular disease
2. Haemorrhage
   a. Significant haemorrhage occurs in approximately 1% of patients undergoing endoscopic polypectomy
   b. Haemorrhage usually stops spontaneously but may occasionally require surgical intervention
3. Intra-colonic explosion
   a. Bowel perparation using mannitol causes a high intra-luminal concentration of hydrogen
   b. Explosions may occur with the use of a diathermy snare

FURTHER READING

Campbell W B, Rhodes M, Kettlewell M G W 1985 Colonoscopy following intraoperative lavage in the management of severe colonic bleeding. Ann R Coll Surg Eng 67: 290–292
Cotton P B, Bowden T A 1986 Gastrointestinal endoscopy and the surgeon. In: Russell R C G (ed) Recent Advances in Surgery, Churchill Livingstone, Edinburgh pp 71–88
Fork F-T 1987 Diagnostic procedures in colo-rectal cancer: barium enema or colonoscopy? or both? Eur J Surg Oncol 13: 147–149
Gillespie P E, Chambers T J, Chan K W, Doronzo F, Morson B C Williams C B 1979 Colonic adenomas – a colonoscopy survey. Gut 20: 240–245
Lindsay D C, Freeman J G, Cobden I, Record C O 1988 Should colonoscopy be the first investigation for colonic disease? Br Med J 296: 167–169
Mortensen N J Mc, Eltringham W K, Mountford R A, Lever J V 1984 Direct vision brush cytology with colonoscopy: an aid to the accurate diagnosis of colonic strictures. Ann R Coll Surg Eng 71: 930–932
Vellacott K D 1986 Early endoscopy for acute lower gastrointestinal haemorrhage. Ann R Coll Surg Eng 68: 243–244
Williams C B 1985 Colonoscopy. Curr Opinion in Gastroenterology 1: 54–59

DIVERTICULAR DISEASE OF THE COLON

Introduction

Although the condition is uncommon in younger age groups more than half the population of the Western World aged over 65 years suffer from diverticular disease of the colon. The disorder most commonly affects the sigmoid colon and women tend to be affected more often than men. In many cases the disease is asymptomatic; fortunately only a small minority will suffer serious complications of the disease and require surgical intervention.

Aetiology and pathogenesis

Low residue diet
↓
Elastosis and contraction of taenia coli
↓
Shortening of colonic length
↓
Increased thickness and inappropriate segmentation of colonic circular muscle
↓
Segmental intra-luminal hypertension
↓
Pulsion diverticula of colonic mucosa

Diverticulosis denotes the presence of colonic diverticula; diverticulitis indicates their inflammation

Treatment of uncomplicated diverticular disease

1. High-residue diet
   a. The gastro-intestinal transit time is prolonged in diverticular disease and the daily stool volume and weight are reduced
   b. Transit is accelerated and faecal volume increased by increasing the amount of non-absorbable dietary fibre
   c. It is recommended that patients take at least 20–25 g of fibre per day which can be taken in the form of:
      (i) fresh fruit and vegetables
      (ii) wholemeal bread and flour
      (iii) natural (unprocessed) wheat or oat bran
2. Bulk laxatives
   These have a similar effect to that of a high residue diet and are useful for patients who are unable to take bran:
   a. methylcellulose (Celevac, Cologel)
   b. ispaghula husk (Fybogel, Isogel, Regulan)
   c. sterculia (Normacol)
3. Anti-spasmodic agents
   a. Intraluminal colonic pressure is abnormally high in patients with diverticular disease
   b. It can be reduced by anti-spasmodic drugs which are sometimes used in symptomatic diverticular disease
   c. They have either an anti-cholinergic or direct muscle relaxant effect:
      (i) anti-cholinergic drugs eg propantheline bromide(Por-Banthine), dicyclomine (Merbentyl)
      (ii) smooth muscle relaxants eg mebeverine hydrochloride (Colofac), peppermint oil (Colpermin)
4. Colonic resection
   Surgical resection of a colonic segment affected by uncomplicated diverticular disease may be required if severe symptoms cannot be adequately controlled by conservative measures

Complications
1. Acute inflammation (acute colonic diverticulitis)
   a. Local peritonitis
   b. Pericolic (diverticular) abscess
   c. Generalised purulent or faecal peritonitis
   Small intestinal obstruction, often due to paralytic ileus, can complicate peritonitis caused by acute diverticulitis
2. Fistula formation
   a. Colo-vesical fistula
   b. Colo-vaginal fistula
   c. Colo-colic fistula
   d. Colo-enteric fistula
   e. Colo-cutaneous fistula
3. Stricture formation and colonic obstruction
   a. This is a rare complication of diverticular disease
   b. Repeated episodes of acute inflammation are followed by increasing fibrosis
   c. Carcinoma must always be excluded
4. Haemorrhage
   a. Also an unusual complication occurring in less than 10% of patients with diverticular disease
   b. Haemorrhage is always intra-luminal and may be very severe

Indications for surgery
1. Failure to control chronic symptoms by adequate medical treatment
2. Recurrent episodes of acute diverticulitis
3. Diverticular (pericolic) abscess
4. Generalised purulent or faecal peritonitis
5. Fistula
6. Colonic stricture
7. Massive haemorrhage

Treatment of complications of diverticular disease
1. Acute diverticulitis with localised peritonitis
   a. Bed rest
   b. Intra-venous fluids
   c. Broad spectrum antibiotics
   d. Naso-gastric intubation and aspiration
2. Diverticular abscess
   a. Under general anaesthetic an incision is made over the fluctuant area to allow drainage of pus
   b. A large drainage tube is inserted to prevent further abscess formation

3. Acute diverticulitis with generalised purulent or faecal peritonitis
   a. Pre-operative preparation should include:
      (i) Intra-venous colloid and crystalloid fluids to treat or prevent hypovolaemia
      (ii) Broad spectrum antibiotics including specific anaerobicidal agents such as metronidazole
      (iii) Naso-gastric intubation and aspiration are important in the management of paralytic ileus
      (iv) Urinary catheterisation and measurement of urine output
   b. Conservative surgical treatment used to be popular but is now rarely indicated:
      (i) Suture of colonic perforation
      (ii) Peritoneal lavage
      (iii) Intra-peritoneal drainage
      (iv) Defunctioning transverse colostomy or caecostomy
      Conservative surgical treatment usually fails to control or eliminate the infective focus in the sigmoid colon and is associated with a high post-operative morbidity and mortality. It is now only indicated in those patients where radical treatment is not feasible
   c. Radical surgical treatment
      Resection of the affected segment of colon, usually the sigmoid, eliminates the source of continuing peritoneal contamination and prevents further systemic absorption of bacteria and bacterial toxins. Such radical treatment is associated with half the operative mortality of conservative procedures and is now regarded as the treatment of choice
      (i) without primary anastomosis
         – Paul–Mickulicz procedure if the distal colonic segment is sufficiently long
         – Formation of terminal colostomy and mucous fistula if a long rectal stump can be preserved
         – Hartmann's procedure if only a short rectal stump is present
      Continuity of the colon can be restored by secondary anastomosis performed approximately 2–3 months later
      (ii) with primary anastomosis
      Intra-operative orthograde colonic irrigation has been used to improve the results of this form of treatment which should only be performed by experienced surgeons
4. Fistulae
   a. Multi-staged resection is usually performed although the first two stages may be combined
      Stage 1: Initial defunctioning colostomy allows inflammation at the site of the fistula to subside

Stage 2: Resection of the diseased colon and fistulous tract with end-to-end colonic anastomosis
   (i) Layered closure of organ involved by the fistula
   (ii) Greater omental interposition to prevent recurrence
Stage 3: Closure of defunctioning colostomy

b. Single-staged resections should not be undertaken in the presence of severe infection or with a patient in poor general health as they are associated with high morbidity and mortality

5. Stricture
   Colonic resection and primary anastomosis
6. Haemorrhage
   a. Blood transfusion is required to treat or prevent hypovolaemic shock
   b. In many patients haemorrhage ceases spontaneously; continued massive haemorrhage requires urgent investigation to localise its source and appropriate surgical treatment
   c. In patients with radiologically proven diverticular disease acute lower gastro-intestinal haemorrhage is often attributable to angiodysplasia, usually of the caecum or ascending colon
   d. Barium enema examination will not localise the source of such bleeding and may make subsequent arteriography difficult
   e. Colonoscopy allows visualisation of the entire colonic mucosa, localisation of the bleeding point and identification of areas of angiodysplasia
   f. Provided active bleeding is occurring at a rate of at least 1.0 ml/min at the time of the examination, arteriography can be used to accurately localise the source of haemorrhage and allow conservative colonic resection
   g. 'Blind' local colonic resection based on the distribution of diverticular disease is associated with a high rate of recurrent haemorrhage
   h. Total colectomy with terminal ileostomy or primary ileorectal anastomosis should only be performed if the source of haemorrhage has not been accurately localised

FURTHER READING

Farrands P A, Taylor I 1987 Management of acute lower gastrointestinal haemorrhage in a surgical unit over a 4-year period. J Roy Soc Med 80: 79–82

Krukowski Z H, Matheson N A 1984 Emergency surgery for diverticular disease complicated by generalised and faecal peritonitis. Br J Surg 71: 921–927

Morris D L, Tudor R G 1987 The management of inflammatory complications of colonic diverticular disease. Br J Hosp Med 37: 36–41

Morrison P D, Addison N V 1983 A study of colovesical fistula in a district hospital. Ann R Coll Surg Eng 65: 221–223

Shephard A A, Keighley M R B 1986 Audit on complicated diverticular disease. Ann R Coll Surg Eng 68: 8–10

Smallwood J A 1982 Diverticular disease: emergency surgical problems. Hosp Update 8: 1554–1561

Vellacott K D 1986 Early endoscopy for acute lower gastrointestinal haemorrhage. Ann R Coll Surg Eng 68: 242–244

Whiteway J, Morson B C 1985 Pathology of ageing – Diverticular disease. Clinics in Gastroenterology 14: 829–846

Whiteway J, Morson B C 1985 Elastosis in diverticular disease of the sigmoid colon. Gut 26: 258–266

ULCERATIVE COLITIS

Ulcerative colitis is a chronic non-specific inflammatory disease of the large intestinal mucosa of unknown aetiology and increasing incidence. The inflammatory process starts distally in the rectum and spreads proximally. Inflammation is confined to the rectum and colon except for occasional 'backwash' terminal ileitis. Differentiation from Crohn's colitis may be difficult.

Pathological features
1. Inflammatory infiltrate and oedema confined to mucosa and submucosa
2. Crypt abscesses
3. Goblet cell depletion
4. Mucosal ulceration
5. Inflammatory pseudo-polyps composed of granulation tissue

Endoscopic features
1. Mucus, blood or pus in colonic or rectal lumen
2. Loss of normal mucosal vascular pattern
3. Mucosal reddening due to hyperaemia or petechial haemorrhages
4. Granular mucosa with contact haemorrhage
5. Mucosal ulceration
6. Pseudo-polyps

Radiological features
1. Colonic dilatation with thickening of the colonic wall on plain abdominal radiographs in toxic megacolon
2. Loss of mucosal definition on barium enema examination with mucosal granularity, ulceration and pseudopolyps
3. Loss of normal haustral pattern

4. Contraction of length and diameter of the colon producing a 'pipe-stem' colon

Local complications
1. Haemorrhage
2. Stricture
3. Carcinoma
4. Acute toxic dilatation of colon (toxic megacolon)
5. Perforation

General complications
1. Arthropathy
2. Episcleritis
3. Aphthous ulceration of mouth
4. Uveitis (iridocyclitis)
5. Ankylosing spondylitis
6. Erythema nodosum
7. Pyoderma gangrenosum
8. Pericholangitis
9. Sclerosing cholangitis
10. Bile duct carcinoma
11. Fatty infiltration of liver
12. Macronodular cirrhosis

Medical management

In remission
1. Oral sulphasalazine (Salazopyrin) reduces the frequency of acute exacerbations; optimum dosage 2 g per day
2. 5-amino salicylic acid (5-ASA) is as effective as sulphasalazine but has fewer side effects as the sulphapyridine moiety is absent; now available as slow-release and enteric coated preparations
3. Codeine phosphate
4. Routine use of systemic steroids is not indicated. Two trials which compared prednisolone 15 mg per day for 6 months and cortisone 25 mg per day for 1 year with placebos showed no reduction in the relapse rate for patients in remission. Higher doses are more likely to maintain remission but the side effects would prevent their routine use
5. Azathioprine (Imuran) may have a steroid-sparing effect in those patients requiring long term steroid therapy
6. Disodium cromoglycate (Nalcrom) was thought to be of some benefit in initial studies but subsequent large scale controlled trials have failed to confirm these findings
7. Nutritional support

In mild attacks
1. Oral sulphasalazine 2 g per day
2. Sulphasalazine enemas
3. Steroid suppositories: prednisolone 5 mg twice daily
4. Steroid retention enemas: prednisolone 20 mg in 100 ml nightly
5. Systemic steroids: oral prednisolone 20–40 mg per day
6. Nutritional support

Response should normally occur within 1–2 weeks and treatment is continued for one month

In severe attacks
A severe acute attack of ulcerative colitis is indicated by the following features:
1. Extreme malaise and weight loss
2. Marked diarrhoea with more than eight bowel actions per day
3. Temperature >38°C and tachycardia
4. Abdominal pain and tenderness
5. Serum albumin below 30 g/l
6. Markedly elevated ESR

Treatment must be energetic and special attention must be directed to the prevention and early recognition of serious complications
   a. Clear fluids only by mouth
   b. Intra-venous fluids, electrolytes and blood transfusion as required
   c. Intensive parenteral nutrition
   d. Systemic steroids: intravenous prednisolone 40–60 mg per day or hydrocortisone 400 mg per day
   e. Broad spectrum antibiotics are commonly used but are of no proven benefit
   f. Daily plain abdominal radiographs are used to assess colonic dilatation and exclude silent perforation

Indications for emergency surgery
1. Deterioration in patient's condition despite adequate medical treatment
2. Failure to show a significant response to adequate medical treatment after 5 days
3. Toxic megacolon
4. Perforation
5. Haemorrhage

Indications for elective surgery
1. Continuous disabling symptoms which fail to respond to adequate medical treatment
2. Persistent complications especially erythema nodosum, pyoderma gangrenosum, uveitis and arthropathy
3. Retardation of growth and development in children

4. Fibrous stricture
5. Colonic carcinoma
6. Severe colonic dysplasia

Emergency surgical procedures
1. Total colectomy, terminal ileostomy and recto-sigmoid mucous fistula
   a. In most cases the rectum can be preserved
   b. Allows a full range of surgical operations to be performed at a subsequent date
2. Panprocto-colectomy and ileostomy
   a. Emergency proctectomy is associated with increased post-operative morbidity
   b. May be required in cases of massive rectal bleeding

Elective surgical procedures
1. Subtotal colectomy and caeco-proctostomy
   a. Now rarely performed
   b. Further surgery is invariably required
2. Total colectomy and ileo-rectal anastomosis
   a. Indicated especially in young patients keen to avoid an abdominal stoma
   b. May be performed as an elective one-stage procedure without a protective ileostomy or as a secondary procedure after total colectomy and formation of mucous fistula
   c. Should only be performed if the rectum is relatively spared of disease and easily distensible
   d. Contraindicated in cases where rectal capacity is small or if there is dysplasia or malignant change within the rectum
   e. Risk of carcinoma developing in the rectal stump is 6% at 20 years and 15% at 30 years
   f. Indefinite regular follow up at 6-monthly intervals with multiple rectal biopsies is required to detect pre-malignant or malignant change
3. Panproctocolectomy with terminal Brooke ileostomy or Koch continent ileostomy
   a. Whole of the large bowel is removed thus curing the patient of inflammatory bowel disease and completely eliminating the risk of malignant change
   b. Peri-muscular excision of the rectum and inter-sphincteric excision of the anal canal minimises impairment of sexual and bladder function
   c. Koch continent ileostomy is constructed with a nipple valve and avoids the need to wear a permanent appliance but it does require regular intubation

   d. The long intra-peritoneal suture line of the Kock ileostomy is
      prone to leakage which may lead to peritonitis or fistula
      formation
   e. Valve failure leads to incontinence of a Kock ileostomy and
      perforation may follow traumatic intubation
4. Total colectomy, mucosal proctectomy and ileo-anal
   anastomosis with ileal reservoir (restorative proctocolectomy)
   a. All diseased mucosa is removed but a permanent stoma is
      avoided
   b. Contraindicated in the presence of severe stenosis or
      fibrosis of the rectum and in those with poor anal sphincter
      function
   c. Only a short rectal muscular cylinder is preserved usually
      extending only 1–2 cm above the pubo-rectalis muscle
   d. Mucosal proctectomy (rectal mucosectomy) is performed
      via the endo-anal approach
   e. Various ileal reservoirs have been designed, e.g. duplicated
      (J) pouch, triplicated (S) pouch, four loop (W) pouch and
      have different functional characteristics
   f. Most patients will void spontaneously but some require
      intermittent catheterisation of the pouch
   g. Complications include pelvic sepsis, anastomotic strictures,
      faecal incontinence and reservoir (pouch) ileitis
   h. A protective ileostomy is used in all cases to reduce the
      incidence and severity of local complications especially
      pelvic sepsis; it can normally be closed after 8–12 weeks
      provided the ileo-anal anastomosis has healed completely

Risk of colorectal carcinoma in ulcerative colitis
Approximately 2% of all patients with chronic ulcerative colitis will
develop a colorectal carcinoma. The diagnosis of colorectal
carcinoma in patients with ulcerative colitis may be difficult
because the lesions are often plaque-like and frequently multiple.
The tumours are often rapidly progressive and the patient may be
incurable at the time of diagnosis. The roles of regular surveillance
and prophylactic surgery are therefore very important.
   Features indicating a patient is at high risk include:
   1. severe first attack
   2. early age of onset
   3. chronic continuous symptoms
   4. extensive or total colitis for more than 10 years
High risk patients should undergo colonoscopic examination at two
yearly intervals. Multiple random biopsies are taken; any
suspicious areas are also biopsied. If severe epithelial dysplasia is
seen prophylactic panproctocolectomy is performed.

FURTHER READING

Badenoch D, Thompson JPS 1983 Surgery for ulcerative colitis. Hosp Update 9: 841–848

Butt J H, Morson B C 1981 Dysplasia and inflammatory bowel disease. Gastroenterology 80: 865–868

Cranley B 1983 The Kock reservoir ileostomy: a review of its development, problems and role in modern surgical practice. Br J Surg 70: 94–99

Dozois R R 1985 Ileal 'J' pouch – anal anastomosis. Br J Surg 72: 580–582

Editorial 1986 Colorectal carcinoma in ulcerative colitis. Lancet ii: 197–198

Hawley P R 1985 Ileorectal anastomosis, Br J Surg 72: S75–6

Lennard-Jones J E 1985 Cancer risk in ulcerative colitis: surveillance or surgery. Br J Surg 72: S84–86

Mortensen N 1988 Spout or pouch? Alternatives for patients with ileostomies. Br Med J 296: 153–154

Nicholls R J, Moskowitz R L, Sheperd N A 1985 Restorative proctocolectomy with ileal reservoir. Br J Surg 72: S76–79

Schofield P F, Manson J M 1986 Indications for and results of operation in inflammatory bowel disease. J R Soc Med 79: 593–595

Truelove S C, Willoughby C P, Lee E C G, Kettlewell M G W 1978 Further experience in the treatment of severe attacks of ulcerative colitis. Lancet ii: 1068

Williams N S, Johnston D 1985 The current status of mucosal proctectomy and ileo-anal anastomosis in the surgical treatment of ulcerative colitis and adenomatous polyposis. Br J Surg 72: 159–168

Williams N S, Johnston D 1985 Mucosal proctectomy and ileo-anal anastomosis. In: Taylor I (ed) Progress in Surgery Vol 1. Churchill Livingstone, Edinburgh pp 95–113

CROHN'S DISEASE

A granulomatous disease of unknown aetiology which may affect any part of the gastro-intestinal tract. Its incidence has been increasing over last 30 years. 30% of all patients have only small intestinal involvement and a further 30% have only large intestinal involvement. The remaining 40% have involvement of both the small and large intestine.

Pathology
1. Transmural inflammation of intestinal wall characterised by the presence of lymphocytes, plasma cells and non-caseating granulomata
2. Mucosal ulceration ranging from small aphthoid ulcers to deep penetrating ulcers
3. Oedema, fibrosis and stricture formation
4. Abscess formation is likely to be followed by the development of fistulae which may involve the skin, bladder, vagina or other parts of the gastro-intestinal tract
5. Regional lymphadenopathy
6. Most patients will relapse after excisional surgery with Crohn's disease at other sites in the gastro-intestinal tract. The

incidence of recurrent disease is related to the length of follow-up; typical recurrence rates are 30–50% at 5 years, 70% at 10 years and 85% at 25 years.

Clinical features
1. Crohn's disease may present as an acute illness with fever abdominal pain and a mass in the right iliac fossa
2. More often the disease has an insidious onset with chronic ill health, diarrhoea, abdominal pain, low grade fever, anaemia, anorexia and weight loss
3. Anaemia is often due to several aetiological factors:
   a. Iron deficiency due to chronic intestinal blood loss
   b. Vitamin B_{12} deficiency following disease or resection of the terminal ileum
   c. Folate deficiency secondary to malabsorption
   d. Toxic bone marrow depression
4. Small intestinal malabsorption leads to malnutrition characterised by weight loss and hypoproteinaemia
5. Protein-losing enteropathy may accentuate the features of malnutrition

Radiological features
Various characteristic features may be evident on plain abdominal radiographs, barium meal and follow through or small bowel tube enema (enteroclysis) and barium enema examinations. In the presence of an entero-cutaneous fistula a fistulogram may give additional information.
1. Mucosal ulceration
   a. Diffuse cobble-stone appearance
   b. Rose-thorn ulcers
2. Separation of adjacent intestinal loops due to mural oedema
3. Narrowing of intestinal lumen due to spasm, oedema and fibrosis (String sign of Kantor)
4. Intestinal dilatation proximal to strictured segments
5. Skip lesions separated by regions of normal intestine
6. Internal and external fistulae

Medical treatment
1. Anti-diarrhoeal agents
   a. Codeine phosphate, loperamide (Imodium) and diphenoxylate with atropine (Lomotil) help control watery diarrhoea
   b. Cholestyramine (Questran) a bile salt chelating agent is useful in treating choloreic diarrhoea caused by the cathartic effects of unabsorbed bile salts on the colonic mucosa
2. Sulphasalazine
   a. Reduces disease activity in patients with large intestinal involvement

   b. No effect in patients with small intestinal Crohn's disease
   c. No evidence to support its use as maintenance therapy
3. Corticosteroids
   a. Significant benefit in acute exacerbations of both small and large intestinal disease
   b. Use is often limited by steroid toxicity
   c. Maintenance therapy has some advantage to patients in remission
4. Azathioprine
   a. May be useful in maintaining a remission
   b. Used in patients with extensive disease for its steroid-sparing action
   c. Should only be used with careful clinical and haematological monitoring and always in doses less than 2.5 mg/kg body weight per day
5. Metronidazole
   a. Useful in patients with persistent perianal sepsis to control anaerobic infection
   b. Long-term use may be complicated by peripheral neuropathy
6. Enteral nutritional support
   a. Vitamin and mineral supplementation
   b. Increased protein-calorie intake
   c. Elemental diets
7. Parenteral nutrition
   a. Used in cases of high output entero-cutaneous fistula or severe malabsorption due to short bowel syndrome
   b. In addition to improving the patient's nutritional state parenteral nutrition may reduce the activity of the Crohn's disease

Local complications
1. Fistulae
   a. Occur in up to 30% of cases the highest incidence being found in ileo-colic disease
   b. Entero-cutaneous fistulae are rarely spontaneous usually occurring after excisional surgery or drainage of an abscess
2. Perianal lesions
   a. Abscesses, fistulae, fissures and other perianal lesions are quite common in Crohn's disease and their incidence is related to the site and extent of the underlying intestinal involvement
   b. Perianal lesions are found in 20–30% of patients with small intestinal disease, 50–60% of those with ileo-colic disease and 70–80% of patients with extensive large bowel Crohn's disease

    c. With the exception of abscesses the perianal lesions associated with Crohn's disease are usually surprisingly painless
3. Stricture leading to intestinal obstruction
4. Abscess
5. Toxic megacolon
6. Perforation
7. Haemorrhage

General complications
1. Biliary calculi
    a. Increased incidence in those patients with terminal ileal disease
    b. Caused by failure of bile salt resorption with reduction in the bile salt pool
2. Urinary calculi
3. Erythema nodosum
4. Pyoderma gangrenosum
5. Uveitis
6. Amyloidosis
7. Arthritis

Indications for emergency surgery
1. Intestinal obstruction
2. Perforation
3. Haemorrhage
4. Colonic dilatation (toxic megacolon)
5. Intra-abdominal abscess
6. Perianal abscess

Indications for elective surgery
1. Chronic perianal suppuration
2. Fistula
3. Subacute intestinal obstruction
4. Chronic disease unresponsive to adequate medical therapy or requiring unacceptably high doses of corticosteroids
5. Persistent anaemia or malnutrition
6. Severe systemic complications such as recurrent polyarthritis, uveitis or pyoderma gangrenosum
7. Growth retardation in children

Surgical management
1. Drainage of abscess
    a. Intra-abdominal
    b. Subcutaneous
    c. Perianal

Simple drainage of an abscess invariably produces a fistula if there is underlying active intestinal disease but spontaneous healing may sometimes occur

2. Strictureplasty
   a. Suitable only for relatively short stricture of the small intestine
   b. The anti-mesenteric border of the narrowed segment is incised longitudinally and closed transversely
3. Stricture dilatation
   a. May be performed using metal bougies or balloon catheters
   b. Short small intestinal strictures are dilated at laparotomy; duodenal and colonic strictures can be dilated endoscopically
4. Excisional surgery (Intestinal resection)
   a. Crohn's disease cannot be cured by excision and it is essential to preserve the maximum length of intestine
   b. The resection margins should be clear of macroscopic Crohn's disease: the presence of microscopic disease does not affect the recurrence rate
   c. Multiple small resections are the preferred method of surgical treatment for multiple short strictures of the small intestine when dilatation or strictureplasty cannot be performed
   d. Resection and primary end-to-end anastomosis is usually possible; limited right hemicolectomy may be performed for ileo-colic disease
   e. Colonic resection and exteriorisation is performed in the presence of marked colonic dilatation, severe sepsis or malnutrition
   f. If indicated, rectal excision should be conservative preserving the perirectal tissues
5. Defunctioning surgery (bypass)
   a. This treatment is not popular at present since disease activity can continue in the bypassed segment with continued morbidity
   b. Anterior gastro-jejunostomy with vagotomy is performed for Crohn's disease of the duodenum where excision would have a high mortality
   c. End-to-side ileo-transverse colostomy is now rarely used to bypass severe disease of the terminal ileum or caecum, excisional surgery being preferred
   d. Split ileostomy or defunctioning colostomy may be indicated as an initial step in patients with severe recto-sigmoid or perianal disease

FURTHER READING

Editorial 1986 The drug treatment of Crohn's disease. Drug Ther Bull
   24: 13–15
Harper P H, Kettlewell M G W, Lee E C G 1982 The effect of split ileostomy
   on perianal Crohn's disease. Br J Surg 69: 608–610
Harrison R A, Clark C G 1986 Conservative surgery in Crohn Disease. In:
   Nyhus L M (ed) Surgery Annual 1986 Vol 18 Appleton-Century-Crofts,
   Norwalk, Connecticut, pp 29–39
Lee E C G, Papaioannou N 1982 Minimal surgery for chronic obstruction in
   patients with extensive or universal Crohn's disease. Ann R Coll Surg Eng
   64: 229–233
Springall R, Thompson J P S 1984 Surgery for Crohn's disease. Hosp
   Update 103: 501–14
Mortensen N J Mc C, Ritchie J K, Hawley P R, Todd I P, Lennard-Jones J E
   1984 Surgery for acute Crohn's colitis: results and long term follow-up. Br
   J Surg 71: 783–784
Alexander-Williams J, Allan A, Morel P, Hawker P C, Dwykes P W, O'Connor
   H 1986 The therapeutic dilatation of enteric strictures due to Crohn's
   disease. Ann R Coll Surg Eng 68: 95–97

COLORECTAL CARCINOMA

Introduction

Colorectal carcinoma remains the second commonest cause of
death from malignant disease. Further improvements in surgical
techniques are unlikely to enhance the survival of patients with
colorectal carcinoma. The main potential for improved survival lies
in the development of efficient screening methods so that patients
present at an earlier stage and in effective forms of adjuvant
therapy.

Screening procedures

Low-risk groups
Testing for faecal occult blood remains the only realistic method for
large scale screening of populations of asymptomatic individuals.
This method has been shown to increase the proportion of
colorectal tumours which are confined to the bowel wall and can be
expected to improve the long-term survival of a screened
population. In addition many adenomatous polyps will also be
detected.

1. All individuals over 40 years should be screened
2. Compliance rate in various studies is between 30 and 50%
3. The Haemoccult II test, an impregnated guaiac slide test, is
   currently favoured as it is relatively cheap and easy to perform
4. Prior to testing patients must take a high roughage, meat-free
   diet for 24 hours

5. Six slides from three consecutive daily bowel movements are tested without rehydration using a peroxidase developer; a blue coloration at 30 seconds indicates a positive test
6. A positive result can be expected in 2–3% of all tests
7. All Haemoccult-positive patients require physical examination, flexible fibre-optic or rigid sigmoidoscopy and double contrast enema or full colonoscopy
8. The Haemoccult test has a sensitivity of 99% and a specificity of 93%
9. The predictive value of a positive test is approximately 20%
10. Repeat testing at 1–2 yearly intervals is probably required

High-risk groups
These include patients with apparently isolated adenomatous polyps, ulcerative colitis, familial adenomatous polyposis and all patients previously treated for adenocarcinoma of the large bowel. Patients with a family history of colorectal cancer or adenomatous polyps are also at increased risk. Regular screening of these patients and their families where relevant should involve double contrast enema examinations, colonoscopy and serial mucosal biopsies if indicated.

1. Adenomatous polyps
   a. It is thought that most colorectal carcinomas arise in adenomatous polyps (the 'adenoma–carcinoma sequence') but only a minority of polyps will become malignant
   b. The malignant potential of adenomatous polyps is governed by their size, histological type and degree of epithelial dysplasia
   c. The incidence of invasive carcinoma in polyps less than 1 cm in diameter is approximately 1%; polyps that are 1–2 cm show a 10% rate of malignancy compared with 50% in those over 2 cm in diameter
   d. The highest malignant potential is seen in villous adenomas where the incidence is about 40%; tubular adenomas have the lowest rate, usually about 5%, whereas adenomas showing both tubular and villous patterns (tubulo-villous adenomas) show an intermediate rate
   e. The malignant potential of all adenomas increases with increasing degrees of epithelial dysplasia
   f. Studies of age distribution curves suggest that the adenoma-carcinoma sequence usually takes more than 5 years and probably averages 10–15 years but in some patients it may take considerably longer than this
2. Ulcerative colitis
   a. The malignant potential of ulcerative colitis is governed by the age at initial presentation, duration of symptoms and the extent of colonic involvement

b. Pre-cancerous epithelial dysplasia may arise in sessile adenomatous polyps but more often it develops in flat mucosa

c. Contrast enema studies therefore have little role in the surveillance of patients with ulcerative colitis

d. Epithelial dysplasia may not be uniform throughout the affected colorectal mucosa; serial rectal biopsies may therefore not accurately predict the degree of dysplasia of the more proximal colonic mucosa

e. Regular colonoscopy, probably at 1–2 yearly intervals, in patients at risk should be combined with multiple colonic biopsies

f. Severe epithelial dysplasia is an indication for procto-colectomy

3. Familial adenomatous polyposis

a. Characterised by the presence of more than 100 adenomas within the large bowel

b. Incidence of 1 in 10,000 of most populations

c. Autosomal dominant inheritance with high penetrance

d. Patients without a family history presumably represent spontaneous genetic mutations

e. Polyps do not usually appear before 10 years of age

f. Adenomatous polyps are present in 90% of sufferers by the age of 25 years

g. By the age of 40 years 90% of untreated patients will have developed at least one carcinoma

h. Asymptomatic patients at diagnosis have a low incidence of carcinoma

i. 50% of symptomatic patients at diagnosis have a carcinoma or develop one within two years

j. Gastric polyps are found in 70% of patients and most patients have polypoid lesions in either the duodenum or jejunum

k. In the absence of a rectal carcinoma treatment usually comprises colectomy and ileorectal anastomosis with careful and regular surveillance of the rectum

l. Total colectomy, mucosal proctectomy and ileo-anal anastomosis with a reservoir is an alternative

m. Screening of all relatives is vitally important

n. Gardner's syndrome is adenomatosis coli plus associated connective tissue tumours such as osteomas, fibromas and desmoid tumours and epidermoid and odontal cysts

Sphincter saving operative procedures for rectal carcinoma

The lymphatic drainage of the rectum is almost exclusively in a proximal direction towards the inferior mesenteric nodes. In addition microscopic spread of the tumour within the wall of the rectum below the lower margin of macroscopically visible tumour is usually minimal and a 2 cm margin is normally acceptable for a curative excision. Sphincter preserving surgery which is potentially curative is therefore theoretically possible in all but those tumours arising in the lowest part of the rectum which are usually best treated by abdomino-perineal excision.

A minority of small rectal tumours may be suitable for curative local excision obviating the need for radical resection and again preserving the anal sphincters.

1. Anterior resection of rectum
   a. Anterior resection was traditionally the sphincter saving procedure for tumours in the upper third of the rectum
   b. Limited access for anastomosis following resection of tumours of the middle third, especially in obese male patients, usually meant that abdomino-perineal excision of the rectum was required
   c. Low anterior resection and anastomosis is now the most popular procedure in these cases, the development of trans-anal circular stapling devices such as the EEA stapling gun having greatly facilitated colorectal anastomosis in these circumstances
   d. In view of the high incidence of anastomotic dehiscence a temporary defunctioning transverse colostomy is often fashioned

2. Abdomino-anal resection
   a. In the Park's endo-anal colo-anal anastomosis the rectum is mobilised as far as the upper part of the anal canal, transected and excised. The colon is passed into the anal canal and using a self-retaining anal retractor a single layer per-anal anastomosis is fashioned between the colon and the dentate line
   b. Pull-through operations are characterised by apposition of the colon and ano-rectal stump by pulling the colon through the anal canal from below
      (i) Babcock–Black operation – following an anal stretch the colon is pulled through the non-everted anorectal stump and any redundant colon is excised 10 days later
      (ii) Maunsell–Weir operation – the colon is pulled through the everted anorectal stump an anastomosis fashioned and the suture line returned to the pelvis
      (iii) Cutait–Turnbull operation – following anal dilatation the colon is drawn through the everted ano-rectal stump and after 10–14 days the excess is excised and the residual colon sutured to the anal canal. The anastomosis either retracts spontaneously or is reduced a few days later

3. Abdomino-sacral (Kraske) operation
   a. Following trans-abdominal mobilisation of the rectum the patient is placed in the lateral position and the rectum approached posteriorly having excised the coccyx

    b. The mobilised colon and rectum are excised and colo-anal anastomosis fashioned

4. Abdomino-trans-sphincteric (York Mason) excision
   a. The rectum is again first mobilised at laparotomy
   b. With the patient placed prone the anal sphincters are divided in the midline posteriorly to allow access to the lower rectum
   c. After excising the rectum end-to-end anastomosis is performed
   d. Accurate apposition of the anal sphincters by their posterior repair results in normal continence

5. Local excision of tumour
   a. Local excision implies removal of the primary tumour with a margin of surrounding normal rectal wall of full thickness but without excising the loco-regional lymph nodes
   b. For successful results patients must be selected according to strict criteria
   c. Tumours should be less than 3 cm in diameter, situated in the lower rectum within 8–10 cm of the anal verge, be either moderately well-differentiated or well-differentiated, and also be mobile and without palpable extra-rectal spread
   d. These selected tumours are likely to be confined to the rectal wall, less than 5% having lymph node metastases
   e. Computed tomographic and radio-isotope scanning have so far failed to offer more direct evidence of nodal status
   f. Several approaches to local excision are available including per-anal, trans-vaginal, posterior (Kraske) approach and the trans-sphincteric (York Mason) approach
   g. Several series have reported 5-year survival rates in excess of 80%

6. Local destruction of tumour
   a. Local tumour destruction is often used as a palliative procedure in patients with evidence of distant metastates or in those patients who are either unfit for or refuse radical surgery
   b. In other selected cases it is the treatment of choice for patients with tumours that meet the criteria for local excision
   c. Endocavity radiotherapy can be performed as an outpatient procedure and without the need for anaesthesia; a 75% 5-year survival rate has been reported in one large series
   d. Electrocoagulation is a readily available technique which is suitable particularly for polypoid lesions but is often associated with bleeding, perforation, and formation of abscesses, fistulae and strictures
   e. Cryotherapy is also associated with significant local morbidity especially stricture formation and haemorrhage but it is claimed that these occur less commonly than with electrocoagulation

    f. External beam megavoltage radiotherapy may provide good palliation for inoperable primary or recurrent tumours with good control of pain, haemorrhage, mucus discharge and tenesmus

    g. Endoscopic resection using a resectoscope has recently been tried in elderly patients who are unfit for major surgery

    h. Laser therapy has been used in obstructing tumours and to reduce bleeding

    i. Intracavity microwave hyperthermia

Surgical techniques designed to reduce local recurrence following excision of colorectal tumours

Mechanical bowel preparation and prophylactic antibiotics and other antimicrobial agents in elective colorectal surgery have made radical resection and primary anastomosis relatively safe procedures. The problem of local tumour recurrence remains. Pelvic recurrence after radical excision is relatively common in tumours of the lower third of the rectum and is explained by anatomical considerations which may may make adequate local excision difficult once the tumour has spread to the perirectal tissues. Local recurrence following restorative resection may in addition be due to inadequate local excision or anastomotic implantation of viable malignant cells. The scope for improvement in surgical techniques is small and mainly involves a consideration of those factors predisposing to local tumour recurrence.

1. Inadequate local clearance
    a. Distal intramural spread of colorectal carcinomas is usually limited to 1 cm
    b. Those few patients with more extensive intramural spread usually have advanced lesions and develop fatal distant metastases before local recurrence becomes evident
    c. A distal clearance of 2 cm is now considered adequate for the majority of rectal tumours
2. Inadequate excision of perirectal tissues
    a. The mesorectum contains an abundance of lymphatic and vascular channels
    b. Deposits of malignant cells have been identified in lymphatic vessels up to 5 cm distal to the lower edge of rectal carcinomas
    c. Complete excision of the mesorectum at the time of anterior resection has reduced the incidence of local recurrence of rectal carcinoma
3. Implantation of exfoliated malignant cells
    a. Large numbers of viable exfoliated malignant cells are present in the bowel lumen adjacent to the sites of colonic transection at the time of excision of large bowel carcinomas

b. Irrigation of the bowel ends with cytotoxic solutions such as mercuric perchloride, chlorhexidine-cetrimide, povidone iodine or sterile water reduces the incidence of local tumour recurrence in uncontrolled series; randomised controlled studies have not been performed

c. Isolation of the segment of colon which contains the tumour using occlusive tapes placed proximal and distal to the tumour has also been advocated

Surgical techniques designed to reduce distant metastases following excision of colorectal tumours

Haematogenous and lymphatic dissemination of tumours cells are the main causes of distant metastases from colorectal tumours. Two surgical techniques have been investigated in an attempt to reduce the incidence of distant metastases.

1. Preliminary ligation of vascular pedicle
   a. Ligation of the vascular pedicle and division of the colon at the elected site of resection before tumour mobilisation, (Turnbull's 'no touch, preliminary isolation technique'), is designed to reduce the risk of haematogenous and lymphatic spread of malignant cells during the operative procedure
   b. Although improved results are claimed when compared with the conventional method of tumour mobilisation followed by pedicle ligation and division of the colon controlled trials have as yet shown no evidence of a beneficial effect
2. High versus low ligation of vascular pedicle
   a. Proximal ligation of the vascular pedicle constitutes a more radical operation than ligation adjacent to the tumour
   b. Retrospective studies have shown no long term survival advantage following curative excision of recto-sigmoid tumours when the inferior mesenteric pedicle is ligated flush with the aorta ('high ligation') compared with more distal ligation ('low ligation')

Adjuvant radiotherapy

Despite improvements in diagnostic, anaesthetic and surgical techniques the overall survival of patients with colo-rectal carcinomas has remained relatively static over many years. However there is now some evidence that adjuvant irradiation may prolong survival and reduce the incidence of local recurrence in some patients. Adjuvant radiotherapy is really only applicable to rectal or recto-sigmoid tumours. It may be given either immediately prior to surgery or at some time after surgery. In some cases it has been given both before and after surgery.

1. Pre-operative radiotherapy
   a. This aims to reduce the number of viable tumour cells thus reducing the risk of disseminating such cells at operation
   b. In addition it may enhance the patient's immune reaction as a result of release of tumour antigens from non-viable tumour cells
   c. Initial trials of pre-operative adjuvant radiotherapy suggested that patients with Dukes' C lesions showed improved survival when compared with control patients
   d. Pre-operative radiotherapy is useful in fixed rectal tumours where the probability of performing a curative resection is low
   e. Most trials have reported no increase in post-operative morbidity or mortality as a result of pre-operative radiotherapy
2. Post-operative radiotherapy
   a. If radiotherapy is given after surgery, patients at high risk, namely those with Dukes' B and C lesions, can be appropriately selected for adjuvant treatment
   b. Patients with intra-peritoneal or hepatic metastases with a poor prognosis would not receive radiotherapy
   c. Patients with Dukes' A tumours in whom surgical cure is possible and local recurrence is improbable are also spared the side effects of radiotherapy
   d. A great disadvantage is that adjuvant treatment cannot start until wound healing is completed and in some cases, especially after abdomino-perineal excision, this may entail a considerable delay

Adjuvant chemotherapy
1. 5-Fluorouracil
   a. Despite several trials which have evaluated different dosage regimens of systemic 5-fluorouracil as a single adjuvant chemotherapeutic agent no statistically significant difference in survival has been shown
   b. Initial results of studies in which 5-fluorouracil is combined with BCG vaccination suggest that adjuvant cytotoxic therapy when combined with immunotherapy may increase patient survival
   c. Adjuvant cytotoxic liver perfusion, injecting 5-fluorouracil into the portal vein via the obliterated umbilical vein at the time of surgery, may reduce the incidence of liver metastates
2. Methyl CCNU plus 5-Fluorouracil
   a. Combination adjuvant chemotherapy may prove more successful than single agent regimens
   b. The combination of methyl CCNU and 5-fluorouracil is currently being investigated

3. Razoxane
   a. Razoxane (Razoxin) interfers with cell division at the G_2M phase
   b. 125 mg twice daily is given for 5 days per week
   c. Treatment is started 4–6 weeks following surgery and continued for 3 years
   d. An increased time to recurrence is seen in patients with Dukes' C carcinomas undergoing apparently curative operations
   e. Acute leukaemia occurs in 3% of patients receiving long-term adjuvant razoxane

Treatment of liver metastases
The presence of liver metastases from a large bowel carcinoma is associated with a poor prognosis. Average survival is only 6 months and most patients if untreated die within 2 years of the diagnosis of hepatic metastases. Various treatment options are available.
   1. Hepatic resection
      a. Patients with a solitary liver metastasis and those with several deposits confined to one lobe may be suitable for surgical resection
      b. Invasion of the portal vein or inferior vena cava preclude surgery which should not be performed if extra-hepatic structures are involved, distant metastases are present or if the primary tumour has recurred
      c. Multiple deposits involving both lobes of the liver are present in over 80% of all patients with liver metastases and are a contraindication to hepatic resection
      d. Patients undergoing resection of solitary liver metastases can expect increased survival
   2. Systemic chemotherapy
      a. Single agents such as 5-fluorouracil are of little if any benefit
      b. Combination chemotherapy using CCNU, 5-fluorouracil, vincristine and streptozotocin produces a complete or partial response in a third of patients but is associated with considerable systemic side effects
      c. Oral urea is without side effects and may improve survival
   3. Radiotherapy
      a. External beam radiotherapy may provide useful palliation of abdominal pain and other symptoms in up to 50% of patients but overall survival is not prolonged
      b. Radiation doses above 35 Gy are liable to produce radiation hepatitis

Other techniques currently being evaluated include hepatic arterial ligation, hepatic arterial embolisation and regional chemotherapy using implantable delivery systems.

FURTHER READING

Editorial 1986 Colorectal carcinoma in ulcerative colitis. Lancet ii: 197–198

Gilbert J M, Hellmann K, Evans M et al 1986 Randomised trial of oral adjuvant razoxane (ICRF 159) in resectable colorectal cancer: five-year follow-up. Br J Surg 73: 446–450

Goldberg S M, Thorson A G 1987 Local therapy of early malignant lesions in the rectum. Eur J Surg Oncol 13: 155–157

Heald R J, Husband E M, Ryall R D H 1982 The mesorectum in rectal cancer surgery – the clue to pelvic recurrence. Br J Surg 69: 613–616

Heald R J, Ryall R D H 1986 Recurrence and survival after total mesorectal excision after rectal cancer. Lancet i: 1479–1482

Hermanek P 1987 Dysplasia-carcinoma sequence, type of adenomas and early colorectal carcinoma. Eur J Surg Oncol 13: 141–143

Killingback M J 1985 Indications for local excision of rectal cancer. Br J Surg 72: S54–56

Lennard-Jones J E 1985 Cancer risk in ulcerative colitis: surveillance or surgery. Br J Surg 72: S84–86

Mann C V 1985 Techniques of local surgical excision for rectal cancer. Br J Surg 72: S57–58

Riddell R H 1985 Dysplasia and cancer in inflammatory bowel disease. Br J Surg 72: S83

Taylor I 1985 Colorectal liver metastases – to treat or not to treat? Br J Surg 72: 511–516

Umpleby H C, Williamson R C N 1987 Anastomotic recurrence in large bowel cancer. Br J Surg 74: 873–878

Williams N S 1984 The rationale for preservation of the anal sphincter in patients with low rectal cancer. Br J Surg 71: 575–581

Winawer S J 1981 Preventive screening and early diagnosis. In: De Cosse J J (ed) Clinical Surgery International: 1. Large Bowel Cancer. Churchill Livingstone, Edinburgh pp 46–62

Urology

BLADDER TUMOURS
Aetiological factors
1. Cigarette smoking
2. Industrial carcinogens
   a. α-naphthylamine
   b. β-naphthylamine
   c. benzidine
3. Schistosomiasis (bilharzia)
4. Chronic inflammation of bladder mucosa
   a. Vesical calculi
   b. Long-term catheterisation
5. Drugs
   a. Cyclophosphamide
   b. Phenacetin

Presentation
1. Haematuria which is often painless
2. Symptoms of cystitis with or without a proven urinary tract infection
3. Positive cytology on routine screening of high-risk patients
4. Microscopic haematuria on routine urinalysis
5. Rarely with symptoms of bladder outflow or ureteric obstruction

Pathology
1. Transitional cell (urothelial) tumours
   a. These are the most common bladder tumours and can appear as papillary, solid or ulcerated lesions at cystoscopy
   b. A purely benign urothelial tumour, often termed a papilloma, is most uncommon; only if the transitional cells covering a lesion are uniform, show minimal mitotic activity and are without an increase in the number of layers can it be classified as a papilloma
   c. In practice all urothelial tumours should be considered as transitional cell carcinomas as this term indicates their potential for malignant behaviour

2. Squamous carcinoma
   a. Metaplastic squamous carcinoma is quite rare
   b. It usually arises in association with chronic irritation of the bladder mucosa as a result of bladder calculi or schistosomiasis
3. Adenocarcinoma
   a. An extremely rare primary tumour
   b. It usually arises at the fundus of the bladder from remnants of the urachus
   c. Adenocarcinomas may also be secondary tumours derived from the large intestine

Staging – TNM classification
Tumour

TIS	Carcinoma in situ (Flat intra-epithelial tumour)	
TA	Papillary tumour confined to epithelium	
T1	Invasion through the basement membrane to the submucosa	
T2	Invasion of superficial muscle	
T3	Invasion of deep muscle	
T4a	Involvement of other pelvic viscera, e.g. prostate, vagina, uterus	
T4b	Involvement of the pelvic or abdominal wall	

[handwritten margin notes: T1 = BM, T2 - SM, T3 DM, T4 V]

Nodes

N0	No evidence of involvement of pelvic lymph nodes
N1	Involvement of a single ipsilateral pelvic lymph node
N2	Involvement of contralateral, bilateral or multiple pelvic lymph nodes
N3	Fixed mass of pelvic lymph nodes separate from the bladder
N4	Involvement of lymph nodes above the pelvic brim

Metastases

M0	No evidence of distant metastases
M1	Distant metastases present

Histological grade

Grade	Histological appearance	Usual macroscopic appearance
Low	Well differentiated	Papillary
Intermediate	Moderately well differentiated	Papillary or solid
High	Poorly differentiated	Solid or ulcerated

Investigation and assessment
Urothelial tumours may arise at multiple primary sites throughout the urinary tract and therefore the whole tract must be examined.

1. Urinalysis and culture to exclude superadded infection including tuberculosis where indicated
2. Intra-venous urography (IVU) to assess upper urinary tracts
3. Chest radiography
4. Cysto-urethroscopy and biopsy
   a. Superficial biopsy using standard biopsy forceps
   b. Larger fragments obtained by trans-urethral resection should include the underlying muscle to allow accurate staging of the tumour
5. Bimanual examination under anaesthesia (EUA) to assess size of tumour and extent of local spread
6. Bipedal lymphangiography to assess lymph node involvement if computed tomography is not available
7. Computed tomography (CT) is now the investigation of choice for accurate staging of invasive bladder carcinomas

Treatment

1. Superficial tumours with no muscle invasion
   a. Biopsy is followed by diathermy electrode coagulation or trans-urethral resection using a diathermy loop
   b. Random biopsies of the adjacent bladder mucosa are taken to exclude carcinoma in situ
   c. Multiple small recurrent tumours can be treated by intra-vesical chemotherapeutic agents such as ethoglucid (Epodyl), triethylenethiophosphoramide (Thiotepa), mitomycin C and doxorubicin (Adriamycin)
   d. Larger multiple lesions can be treated initially by the hydrostatic pressure technique (Helmstein cystodistension)
   e. Cystectomy is occasionally indicated for multiple superfical tumours or multifocal carcinoma in situ
2. Tumour with superficial muscle invasion
   a. Trans-urethral resection (TUR) using a diathermy loop
   b. Partial cystectomy is rarely performed but may be indicated for urothelial tumours arising in diverticula and adenocarcinomas arising from the urachus; in both these sites TUR is not feasible
3. Tumour with deep muscle and perivesical tissue invasion.
      The treatment of T3 tumours remains controversial. The overall survival of these patients is approximatley 30–40% at 5 years and the various treatment options provide very similar results. Recent studies suggest that patients under 65 years are best served by pre-operative radiotherapy and elective cystectomy whereas those over 65 years should receive radical radiotherapy and salvage cystectomy if necessary.
   a. Trans-urethral resection followed by radical radiotherapy is usually associated with less morbidity than cystectomy but radiation cystitis and proctitis may prove troublesome

b. Radical cystectomy plus urinary diversion has a significant operative mortality especially in elderly patients and may be accompanied by considerable morbidity, including impotence in men

c. Radical radiotherapy followed by salvage cystectomy if primary tumour regression is incomplete or if tumour recurrence occurs spares many patients the ordeal of cystectomy and urinary diversion

d. Integrated radiotherapy and cystectomy is associated with significant pre-operative down-staging of the tumour in some patients and in these there may be a slight benefit to patient survival

e. Prophylactic urethrectomy should be performed at the time of cystectomy in patients with multifocal carcinomas

f. Other patients require careful and regular urethroscopic surveillance

4. Tumour invading the pelvic viscera or the pelvic side wall. For T4 tumours treatment is only palliative

a. Haematuria can often be controlled by trans-urethral resection or diathermy coagulation of the intravesical tumour

b. Palliative radiotherapy, cystodistension or intra-vesical formalin are alternatives

c. Occasionally internal iliac artery ligation or therapeutic embolisation is required

d. Appropriate antibiotics should be given if urinary infection is present

e. Urinary frequency may be improved by anti-cholinergic drugs such as propantheline, flavoxate and oxybutynin

f. Palliative supravesical urinary diversion is indicated in very few cases

g. Systemic chemotherapy may be appropriate in some cases but it is thought to be of little value in most

Prognosis

Prognosis is largely determined by the stage of the bladder tumour at presentation

Stage	5-year survival (%)
TA	90–100
T1	70
T2	55
T3	35
T4	10–20

FURTHER READING

Bullock N 1986 Asymptomatic microscopical haematuria. Br Med J 292: 645

Hall R R 1983 Bladder cancer. Hosp Update 9: 317–324

Hendry W F 1986 Morbidity and mortality of radical cystectomy (1971–78 and 1978–85). J R Soc Med 79: 395–400

Herr H W, Landone V P, Whitmore W F 1987 Overview of intravesical therapy for superficial bladder tumours. J Urol 138: 1363–1368

Hunt M T, Woodhouse C R J 1987 Cost-effectiveness of investigations for invasive bladder cancer. J R Soc Med 80: 143–144

Gillatt D A, O'Reilly P H 1987 Haematuria analysed – a prospective study. J R Soc Med 80: 559–560

Woodhouse C R J 1982 Microscopic haematuria. Br J Hosp Med 27: 163–168

PROSTATIC CARCINOMA

Introduction
Prostatic carcinoma is the commonest neoplasm of the male genito-urinary tract and the fourth commonest malignancy in men. It becomes more common with increasing age. Although frequently giving rise to symptoms it is often an incidental finding at postmortem examination in elderly men dying as a result of other causes.

Staging – TNM classification
Tumour
T0   No tumour palpable: Incidental finding in operative specimen or transurethral resection prostatic chippings.
T1   Intra-capsular tumour surrounded by normal prostatic tissue.
T2   Intra-capsular tumour distorting the surface of the prostate gland.
T3   Extra-capsular spread of tumour.
T4   Tumour invading adjacent structures or fixed to pelvic wall.
Nodes
N0   No lymph node involvement.
N1   Single lymph node involved below the iliac bifurcation.
N2   Multiple lymph nodes involved below the iliac bifurcation.
N3   Fixed nodal mass on pelvic side wall.
N4   Common iliac and para-aortic lymph nodes involved.
Metastases
M0   No evidence of distant metastases.
M1   Distant metastases present.

Diagnosis
1. Histological examination of fragments of prostatic tissue resected endoscopically or removed at open prostatectomy

2. Tru-Cut needle biopsy
   a. Trans-rectal biopsy
   b. Trans-perineal biopsy
3. Aspiration cytology

Investigations
1. Serum acid phosphatase (phospho-monoesterase II)
2. Intra-venous urography (IVU)
3. Isotope bone scintigraphy
4. Radiographic skeletal survey
5. Bipedal lymphangiography
6. Computed tomography
7. Trans-rectal ultrasonography

The first four investigations are used routinely in the assessment and staging of patients with prostatic carcinoma. If available computed tomography is generally preferred to lymphangiography in assessing the pelvic lymph nodes.

Treatment of localised disease
1. Trans-urethral resection of prostate (TURP)
2. Radiotherapy
   a. External beam radiotherapy to the prostate is indicated in young patients who have no evidence of bony metastases
   b. Pelvic lymph nodes are usually included in the therapeutic fields
   c. Complications include radiation cystitis and proctitis and urethral stricture
3. Radical prostatectomy
   a. Although not favoured in the UK this operation is popular in the USA where it is usually combined with pelvic lymphadenectomy
   b. Should only be performed in patients with small tumours localised to the prostate
   c. Impotence was inevitable and incontinence occurred in up to 50% of patients but since the development of the nerve sparing technique both these complications are now much less common

Hormonal manipulation in the treatment of disseminated disease
Almost one half of all patients with prostatic carcinoma have metastatic disease at the time of presentation. Androgen suppression or use of specific androgen antagonists will produce symptomatic relief in disseminated prostatic carcinoma in up to 75% of patients. Hormonal manipulation is most effective when first used but has no effect on long-term survival in patients with asymptomatic metastases. Therefore most patients do not receive hormonal manipulation at the time of diagnosis. It is only commenced at a later date when patients with disseminated disease become symptomatic.

1. Surgical castration
   a. Bilateral total or subcapsular orchidectomy abolishes testicular androgen secretion and reduces the circulating androgen levels by 95%
   b. Impotence occurs in all patients and hot flushes are seen in 20% of orchidectomised patients
2. Oestrogen therapy
   a. Diethylstilboestrol 1–3 mg per day also reduces circulating testosterone levels
   b. Painful gynaecomastia, impotence, testicular atrophy and salt and water retention with ankle oedema are commonly seen
   c. More important side effects which include hypertension, myocardial infarction, cerebro-vascular accidents, deep vein thrombosis and pulmonary embolism have been shown to increase mortality
3. Cyproterone acetate (Cyprostat)
   a. A steroid androgen antagonist which inhibits growth of androgen dependent prostatic carcinomas
   b. Progestogenic activity inhibits gonadotrophin release producing a fall in circulating testosterone levels
   c. Given orally in a dose of 100 mg 8–12 hourly
   d. May be used following orchidectomy to prevent hot flushes
4. Flutamide
   a. A non-steroidal pure androgen antagonist
   b. Has fewer side effects than oestrogens but the control of the disease is no better and in some cases may be worse
5. Aminoglutethimide (Orimetin)
   a. Prevents adrenal androgen secretion
   b. Is used in advanced prostatic carcinoma and symptomatic relief may occur in up to 50% of cases
   c. Often causes lethargy and somnolence
   d. Corticosteroid replacement therapy is essential
6. Leuteinising hormone releasing hormone (LHRH) agonists
   a. LHRH is a decapeptide produced by the hypothalamus which causes release of leuteinising hormone (LH) from the anterior pituitary gland. This in turn stimulates testicular secretion of testosterone
   b. LHRH agonists cause down regulation of the hypophyseal LHRH receptors producing a fall in LH secretion with consequent reduction in testosterone secretion by the testes
   c. After an initial rise in serum testosterone concentration, serum testosterone levels fall to those seen following surgical castration after 2–4 weeks
   d. Goserelin (Zoladex), a synthetic analogue of the naturally occurring hypothalamic LHRH, is given by subcutaneous injection at monthly intervals

e. Clinical response rates are similar to those seen after orchidectomy; hot flushes, decreased libido and impotence occur to the same extent with the two forms of therapy

f. Cyproterone acetate may be required temporarily following the first injection of an LHRH agonist to control increased symptoms which are seen in about one third of patients and are due to the initial rise of serum testosterone

Radiotherapeutic treatment of disseminated disease
1. External beam radiotherapy is used to treat symptomatic skeletal metastases
2. ^{32}P phosphorus has been used to treat widespread bony metastases

Cytotoxic chemotherapy
1. Single agent chemotherapy using drugs such as cyclophosphamide, 5-flourouracil and melphalan has proved of little value in treating prostatic carcinoma which does not respond to hormonal manipulation or has recurred following a previous successful response
2. Combination chemotherapy with adriamycin and methotrexate with subsequent folinic acid rescue may prove useful
3. Estramustine phosphate (Estracyt) is phosphorylated oestradiol linked to a nitrogen mustard reported to produce benefit in half of all patients in one trial

Prognosis
1. Patients with small primary lesions without metastatic disease (T0–T1, N0, M0) have a 70–75% 10-year survival
2. Larger primary lesions (T2–T3) are associated with a 50% 5-year survival
3. Patients with metastatic disease (M1) have a 25% 5-year survival and a 10% 10-year survival

FURTHER READING

Editorial 1986 Management of metastatic prostatic carcinoma. Drug Ther Bull 24: 85–88
Editorial 1985 Dilemmas in the management of prostatic carcinoma. Lancet ii: 1219–20
Grant J B F, Ahmed S R, Shalet S M, Costello C B, Howell A, Blacklock N J 1986 Testosterone and gonadotrophin profiles in patients on daily or monthly LHRH analogue ICI 118630 (Zoladex) compared with orchiectomy. Br J Urol 58: 539–544
Kirk D 1987 Trials and tribulations in prostatic cancer. Br J Urol 59: 375–379
Linholt J, Hansen P T 1986 Prostatic carcinoma: complications of megavoltage radiation therapy. Br J Urol 58: 52–54

Parmar H, Phillips R H, Lightman S L, Edwards L, Allen L, Schally A V 1985
    Randomised controlled study of orchidectomy versus long-acting D-Trp-
    6-LHRH microcapsules in advanced prostatic cancer. Lancet ii: 1201–1205
Rickards D, Gowland M, Broodman P, Mamtora H, Blacklock N J, Isherwood
    I 1983 Computed tomography and transrectal ultrasound in the diagnosis
    of prostatic disease – a comparative study. Br J Urol 55: 726–732
Smedley H M, Sinnott M, Freedman L S, Macaskill P, Naylor C P E, Pillers
    E M K 1983 Age and survival in prostatic carcinoma. Br J Urol
    55: 529–533
Walsh P C, Mostwin J L 1984 Radical prostatectomy and
    cystoprostatectomy with preservation of potency. Results using a new
    nerve sparing technique. Br J Urol 56: 694–697
Waxman J 1987 Gonadotrophin hormone releasing analogues open new
    doors in cancer treatment. Br Med J 295: 1084–1085

METHODS OF URINARY DIVERSION

Introduction
The methods of urinary diversion may be classified as follows:
1. Temporary or permanent
2. Intubated or non-intubated
3. Vesical or supra-vesical

Nephrostomy
1. Drainage via a simple catheter inserted into an obstructed
   kidney is only suitable as a method of short term urinary
   diversion
2. Drainage tubes may be inserted at operation or percutaneously
   under ultrasound or radiologiocal control
3. Loop nephrostomy is useful where more prolonged drainage is
   required; a new tube is easily inserted using a railroading
   technique

Ureterostomy in situ
1. A convenient form of temporary urinary diversion useful in
   emergency situations such as bilateral lower ureteric
   obstruction and often preferable to nephrostomy drainage
2. A catheter is inserted into the unmobilised ureter just above
   the pelvic brim and advanced into the renal pelvis
3. Once a tract has formed the catheter can be changed easily
4. Often a simpler alternative to insertion of a nephrostomy tube
   at open operation and is therefore a preferred technique

Loop cutaneous ureterostomy
1. Can be used to provide temporary urinary diversion in
   neonates or small infants with advanced hydro-ureter and
   hydro-nephrosis caused by lower urinary tract obstruction
2. The loop is constructed from the dilated tortuous ureter as
   close as possible to the pelvi-ureteric junction to provide
   effective decompression of the obstructed kidneys

End cutaneous ureterostomy
1. A ureter of normal calibre can seldom be exteriorised at an optimal site; in addition there is a marked tendency to stenosis at the uretero-cutaneous junction
2. Skin flaps can be used to construct a spout and to prevent stomal stenosis
3. Ureters which are grossly dilated often have sufficient length to be exteriorised at a single site as a double-barrelled stoma
4. Conversion to ileal conduit diversion can be performed at a later date if necessary

Transuretero-ureterostomy
1. Indicated for conditions involving the distal ureter in the presence of a normal contralateral ureter
2. Provides an alternative to a psoas hitch with ureteric reimplantation or the Boari bladder flap uretero-cystoplasty
3. Contraindicated where ureteric obstruction is due to malignant disease or irradiation stricture

Suprapubic cystostomy
1. Indicated in cases of bladder outflow obstruction, urethral trauma and stricture
2. Catheter can be inserted percutaneously or at open operation
3. A small diameter catheter inserted obliquely through the anterior abdominal wall minimises leakage of urine around the catheter
3. Catheter must be changed regularly and the bladder irrigated at frequent intervals to prevent calculus formation

Cutaneous vesicostomy
1. The bladder is marsupialised either directly or using a bladder flap to provide surface drainage of urine onto the anterior abdominal wall
2. Is used in infants with urethral valves
3. Residual urine in the bladder may lead to infection and calculus formation

Isolated ileal conduit
1. The most popular method of permanent urinary diversion in both adults and children and now the preferred technique in most cases
2. Either a short transperitoneal segment or a longer extraperitoneal segment of ileum can be used
3. The peristaltic activity of the ileum is greater than that of the colon and ensures rapid emptying of the conduit thus preventing urinary stasis, bacterial overgrowth and retrograde urinary infection

4. Anti-reflux techniques are not usually used at the uretero-ileal anastomoses as they are important only for reservoirs and not conduits
5. The stoma of the ileal conduit should be constructed away from bony prominences, the umbilicus, skin creases and scars to allow proper fitting of the collecting appliance
6. Complications include stenosis at the uretero-ileal anastomosis, stenosis and retraction of the stoma and calculus formation within the conduit

Continent urinary reservoir
1. A low pressure reservoir is essential to prevent deterioration in renal function
2. The reservoir is emptied by intermittent self-catheterisation
3. Examples include the continent ileal reservoir (Koch pouch) and the Mainz ileo-caecal reservior
4. The Penn pouch involves application of the Mitrofanoff principle in which the appendix is used as the route of catheterisation of an ileo-caecal reservoir

Uretero-sigmoidostomy
1. Prior to the development of the isolated colon and ileal conduits uretero-sigmoidostomy was the method of choice for permanent urinary diversion following cystectomy
2. Serious complications occurred in almost 50% of patients
   a. Ascending urinary infection leading to acute and chronic pyelonephritis
   b. Hyperchloraemic, hypokalaemic acidosis
   c. Incontinence of liquid stool in cases with poor anal sphincter function
3. Conversion to an isolated colon conduit or a rectal bladder is considered if the complications cannot be controlled
4. Uretero-colic anastomoses predispose to the development of adenomatous colonic polyps and adenocarcinomas which are most common in the immediate vicinity of the ureteric orifices
5. A latent period of 20–25 years between diversion and neoplasia is usually seen and regular surveillance must be continued indefinitely

Isolated colon conduit
1. External colonic loop urinary diversion does not appear to carry the same carcinogenic risk as uretero-sigmoidostomy and is not usually associated with any electrolyte disturbances
2. Because of the greater diameter of the colon and the wider stoma that is fashioned the incidence of stomal stenosis is less than that with ileal conduits

3. Following pelvic exenteration for recurrent pelvic neoplasms an isolated colon conduit formed from the sigmoid colon distal to a descending colostomy has the advantage of avoiding an intestinal anastomosis

Rectal bladder

1. The ureters are implanted into the upper rectum which is closed off and a terminal sigmoid colostomy fashioned
2. Can be performed as a primary procedure (primary rectal bladder) or by conversion of a uretero-sigmoidostomy in cases where there is severe hyperchloraemic acidosis or ascending pyelonephritis (secondary rectal bladder)
3. Almost the whole length of both ureters must be preserved for anastomosis to the rectum without tension: formation of a bladder from the recto-sigmoid rather than the rectum alone increases its capacity and is indicated when shorter lengths of ureter are available
4. Good anal sphincter function is essential
5. No intestinal anastomosis is involved

FURTHER READING

Ashken M H 1987 Stomas continent and incontinent. Br J Urol 59: 203–207
Boyd S D, Skinner D G, Lieskovsky G 1987 The continent ileal reservoir (Kock pouch). Seminars in Urology 5: 15–27
Duckett J W, Snyder H M 1986 Continent urinary diversion: variations of the Mitrofanoff principle. J Urol 136: 58–62
Duckett J W, Snyder H M 1987 The Mitrofanoff principle in continent urinary reservoirs. Seminars in Urology 5: 55–57
Hill J T, Ransley P G 1983 The colonic conduit: a better method of urinary diversion. Br J Urol 55: 629–631
Stewart M 1986 Urinary diversion and bowel cancer. Ann R Coll Surg Eng 68: 98–102
Stewart M, Macrae F, Williams C B 1982 Neoplasia and ureterosigmoidoscopy – colonoscopy survey. Br J Surg 69: 414–416
Thuroff J W, Alken P, Englemann U et al 1986 The Mainz pouch (mixed augmentation of ileum and caecum applicable for bladder augmentation/substitution and continent urinary diversion). J Urol 136: 17–26

TRAUMA TO THE URINARY TRACT

Mechanisms

1. Non-penetrating injury
   a. Blunt trauma,
      e.g. to kidney, full bladder or perineal urethra
   b. Deceleration injury,
      e.g. to kidney and proximal ureter

2. Penetrating injury,
   e.g. stab or missile injuries and penetration of the lower urinary
   tract by fragments from a pelvic fracture
3. Indirect trauma,
   e.g. disruption of symphysis pubis causing urethral injury
4. Iatrogenic injury,
   e.g. damage to ureters or bladder during laparoscopy, pelvic or
   trans-urethral surgery and urethral trauma during
   catheterisation

Investigations
1. Plain abdominal and pelvic radiographs.
   Abnormalities include:
   a. Loss of psoas shadow due to retroperitoneal haematoma
   b. Lower rib fractures
   c. Fractured lumbar transverse processes
   d. Displacement of colon by large haematoma
   e. Pelvic fractures, especially disruption of the symphysis
      pubis
2. Intra-venous urogram (IVU).
   All patients with macroscopic haematuria following suspected
   urinary trauma should have an emergency intra-venous
   urogram not only to define the nature, site and extent of the
   injury but to confirm the presence of a normally functioning
   kidney on the contralateral side. In cases of mild injury an
   entirely normal IVU may be obtained. Abnormalities which
   may be seen following moderate or severe trauma include:
   a. Calyceal damage
   b. Extravasation of contrast medium
   c. Filling defects in the pelvi-calyceal system and ureter due to
      blood clot
   d. Indistinct renal outline
   e. Non-visualisation of part of the pelvi-calyceal system
   f. Delayed renal opacification or total non-opacification
3. Urethro-cystography.
   May be useful in the early management of urethral trauma
   demonstrating the site and extent of a urethral or bladder
   injury. Introduction of infection is a potential hazard
4. Urethrography.
   Can be used to detect urethral trauma soon after injury but
   infection is again a possible complication and the procedure
   must always be performed under strict aseptic conditions.
   Later on urethrography or urethroscopy may be used to
   demonstrate post-traumatic urethral strictures
5. Renal arteriography.
   Urgent indications for arteriography include the presence of an
   expanding haematoma in the loin and features suggestive of
   severe renal injury on the emergency intra-venous urogram

associated with with signs of continued haemorrhage. Later indications include macroscopic haematuria persisting more than one week after injury, suspicion of a traumatic arterio-venous fistula and hypertension. Abnormal findings include:
  a. Renal cortical lacerations with extravasation of contrast
  b. Non-filling of all or part of the renal vasculature due to damage to major or minor vessels
  c. Arterio-venous fistula
  d. Cortical atrophy
6. Radio-isotope scintigraphy.
   An alternative method of demonstrating reduced blood flow to part of the kidney or complete renal devascularisation
7. Ultrasound scan.
   Serial scans are used to assess an expanding haematoma
8. Computed tomography.
   Serial measurements are again useful to assess any change in size of a renal mass

Kidney

During laparotomy for associated intra-peritoneal injuries a perinephric haematoma should not be explored unless it is increasing in size. Haemorrhage has usually stopped by the time of surgery due to the tension caused by the haematoma within the retroperitoneum. Relase of this tension caused by exploration of the haematoma allows further bleeding and may necessitate nephrectomy.
1. Trauma to the renal substance rarely requires surgery; the following are indications for exploration of a kidney:
   a. Haemorrhage from a penetrating wound of the kidney
   b. Signs of progressive haemorrhage which may be associated with an enlarging perirenal mass
   c. Continued massive haematuria of renal origin
   d. Drainage of extravasted urine
   e. Infected haematoma
2. Immediate exploration of a damaged kidney should be via a trans-peritoneal approach to allow control of the renal artery and vein prior to exposure of the kidney. A full laparotomy can be performed and damage to the intra-peritoneal contents assessed but problems with urinary fistulae may occur later
3. Delayed exploration is via a standard loin incision as a complete laparotomy is not required at this stage
4. A perinephric haematoma and any extravasated urine are drained
5. Lacerations of the renal substance and tears of the renal pelvis are repaired
6. Polar or partial nephrectomy is sometimes possible if part of the kidney is severely damaged or devascularised

7. Nephrectomy may be indicated for a severely traumatised kidney provided a functioning kidney is present on the contralateral side

8. Avulsion injuries in which the renal pedicle is torn may be suitable for treatment by replantation of the devascularised kidney in the contralateral iliac fossa

9. All patients who have suffered renal trauma must be carefully followed for at least one year as they may develop ureteric obstruction or hypertension

10. Surgery may be required at a later date for reno-vascular hypertension, hydronephrosis or for persistent haematuria which is usually due to an arterio-venous fistula

Ureter
Damage to the ureters is usually iatrogenic but it may ocassionally be caused by a penetrating injury. Iatrogenic ureteric injury is usually associated with technically difficult pelvic operations for sepsis or carcinoma and especially for recurrent carcinoma or after radiotherapy. Ureteric injuries are sometimes identified immediately they are produced. In these cases immediate repair should be carried out. Other injuries present in the early post-operative period usually as a urinary fistula. An IVU and retrograde ureterogram if required are performed and early correction is usually recommended. In some cases repair is performed at a later date.

1. Incomplete injuries which do not involve loss of continuity of the ureter such as inadvertent ligation or crushing may be treated by removal of the ligature, if still present, and insertion of a ureteric catheter

2. Diathermy coagulation may be a more serious injury requiring excision of part of the ureter

3. For ureteric injuries above the pelvic brim associated with loss of length of less than 2 cm primary anastomosis of the spatulated ends may be performed

4. For injuries with more extensive loss of ureteric length a transuretero-ureterostomy is required; auto-transplantation of the kidney to the contralateral iliac fossa is a possible alternative

5. If the ureter is injured below the pelvic brim re-implantation into the bladder using an anti-reflux technique is performed; re-implantation may be facilitated by a psoas hitch or Boari flap

Bladder
Damage may occur with blunt trauma to a distended bladder or in association with a pelvic fracture. Perforation of the bladder may also occur at the time of cystodiathermy or trans-urethral resection of bladder tumours.

1. Intra- and extra-peritoneal perforations should be explored at laparotomy and closed; adequate drainage is essential
2. Urethral or suprapubic catheter drainage is required for 2 weeks following repair of the injured bladder
3. Small iatrogenic extra-peritoneal perforations of the bladder or prostatic capsule occurring at trans-urethral surgery can usually be treated conservatively by catheter drainage provided a large volume of irrigating fluid has not escaped into the retroperitoneal tissues
4. Vesico-vaginal fistula, a complication of hysterectomy or more rarely prolonged obstructed labour, can be corrected by an abdominal approach. A full thickness of bladder wall and vaginal wall are mobilised at the site of the fistula and each closed separately. A buttress of pedicled omentum may used to separate the two suture lines and to provide additional vasculature

Urethra
Urethral injury is far more common in men than women. The short female urethra is rarely traumatised. The anatomical site of injury is not always obvious.

Bulbous urethra
The bulbar urethra is most commonly damaged from within by passage of a cystoscope or urethral catheter. More serious disruption injury usually results from direct perineal trauma, the urethra being crushed against the symphysis pubis.
1. A large haematoma or any extravasated urine should be drained but attempts at primary repair of the urethral tear should not be made
2. One careful attempt at passage of a soft, narrow blunt-ended urethral catheter by an experienced surgeon may succeed in draining the bladder and is unlikely to convert a partial tear into a complete one
3. A suprapubic cystostomy is performed in those cases where urethral catheterisation is unsuccessful. After 10–14 days the patients undergoes panendoscopy and full urological assessment
4. If this examination is satisfactory the suprapubic catheter is clamped and the patient is allowed an attempt to void urine per urethram
5. Any subsequent urethral stricture can be managed by intermittent dilatation, urethrotomy or urethroplasty

Membranous urethra
Injuries of the membranous urethra may be associated with pelvic fractures in which there is disruption of the pelvic ring involving separation of the pubis from the ischial rami. They are more

serious than bulbar urethral injuries and should always be suspected in a patient with a pelvic fracture who is unable to pass urine but has bleeding from the external urinary meatus. As with the management of injuries to the bulbar urethra considerable controversy surrounds the management of those of the membranous urethra. The main object of surgical treatment is to minimise the incidence and severity of subsequent urethral stricture formation and to avoid infection.

1. There is always a possibility that passage of a urethral catheter may cause further damage to the traumatised urethra
2. Failure to successfully pass a catheter into the bladder per urethram necessitates formal suprapubic drainage. Exploration may also exclude any coexistent bladder injury
3. Protagonists of early repair believe that membranous urethral injury is usually complete with some degree of prostatic displacement, a situation which makes future urethroplasty difficult unless realignment is achieved
4. At suprapubic exploration a urethral catheter is passed up the urethra into the prostatic urethra under direct vision to achieve correct alignment of the urethra
5. The alignment and apposition of the prostate with the pelvic floor is then maintained by sutures; traction on the urethral catheter may cause damage to the urinary sphincters
6. The retropubic space is drained; urinary drainage is provided by a separate suprapubic catheter
7. The opposing view is that injuries of the membranous urethra are usually incomplete and that any instrumentation may convert a partial tear into a complete one
8. Suprapubic catheterisation is necessary if urethral catheterisation is not attempted
9. The damaged urethra is then examined by urethroscopy 2–3 weeks after the initial injury and where possible a urethral catheter inserted
10. If complete separation of the prostatic and membranous urethras has occurred and the injury has been treated solely by suprapubic cystostomy repair after some delay may be extremely difficult: for this reason primary repair is usually favoured for all membranous urethral injuries provided the patient's general condition is satisfactory

FURTHER READING

Bewes P 1983 Open and closed abdominal injuries. Br J Hosp Med 29: 402–410
Mundy A R 1985 Urinary tract injuries. Hosp Update 11: 115–122

TESTICULAR TUMOURS

Although rare, accounting for less than 1% of all male cancers, testicular tumours are increasing in incidence. The factors responsible for the substantial increase in recent years remain uncertain.

Introduction
1. Germ-cell tumours account for almost 90% of all malignant neoplasms of the testis
2. They tend to occur in the age range 20–40 years and their overall incidence has been increasing over the last few years
3. Of the two main tumours seminoma tends to occur at later age than teratoma
4. Seminoma tends to present at an earlier stage, is more radiosensitive and has a better prognosis than teratoma which has a much greater metastatic potential
5. Other malignant testicular tumours include lymphomas, mesenchymal tumours and Sertoli cell tumours
6. The testes may also be the site of leukaemic deposits especially in relapse following treatment

Classification of germ-cell tumours
1. Teratoma (35%)
   a. Teratoma differentiated (TD)
      'teratoma' – 5%
   b. Malignant teratoma intermediate (MTI)
      'teratocarcinoma' – 55%
   c. Malignant teratoma undifferentiated (MTU)
      'embryonal carcinoma' – 35%
   d. Malignant teratoma trophoblastic (MTT)
      'choriocarcinoma' – 5%
2. Seminoma (50%)
   a. Classical
   b. Spermatocytic
   c. Anaplastic
3. Mixed seminoma–teratoma (15%)

Staging (Royal Marsden Hospital staging system)
Stage I: No evidence of metastatic disease
Stage II: Involvement of infra-diaphragmatic lymph nodes
   II A – metastases < 2 cm diameter
   II B – metastases 2–5 cm diameter
   II C – metastases > 5 cm diameter
Stage III: Involvement of infra- and supra-diaphragmatic lymph nodes

Infra-diaphragmatic lymph nodes
A, B and C as for Stage II
Supra-diaphragmatic lymph nodes
M – mediastinal lymph nodes
N – cervical lymph nodes
Stage IV: Extra-lymphatic metastases
H – hepatic metastases
L – pulmonary metastases
L1 – less than three small metastases (<2 cm diameter)
L2 – multiple small metastases (<2 cm diameter)
L3 – multiple large metastases (>2 cm diameter)

Investigations
1. Tumour markers
   a. 70% of teratomas produce alpha fetoprotein (AFP), 60% secrete human chorionic gonadotrophin (HCG); almost 90% of all teratomas produce one or other of these markers
   b. All choriocarcinomas secrete HCG but non produce AFP
   c. Less than 10% of seminomas secrete HCG whereas none produce AFP
   d. Other tumour markers currently being evaluated include lactate dehydrogenase (LDH), human placental lactogen (HPL) and placental alkaline phosphatase (PLAP)
2. Chest radiography
3. Whole lung tomography is only required if computed chest tomography is not available
4. Bipedal lymphangiography used to be the only method of assessing the retroperitoneal lymph nodes; with the advent of ultrasonography and computed tomography it is now only used if these investigations have failed to show enlarged lymph nodes
5. Abdominal ultrasonography is used to detect hepatic metastases
6. Abdominal and chest computed tomography

Treatment of seminoma
1. Orchidectomy
   a. Through an inguinal incision the testis is delivered, its cord having been previously clamped at the internal ring to prevent intra-vascular dissemination of tumour
   b. Exploration of a testis through a scrotal incision allows the tumour to spread to the inguinal lymph nodes and in addition favours recurrence of the disease within the scrotum
   c. Surveillance at regular intervals of one to three months for Stage 1 disease is currently favoured, more than 75% of patients requiring no further treatment

2. Radiotherapy
    a. A policy of routine surveillance for Stage I patients is currently being studied with a view to replacing the conventional adjuvant treatment of para-aortic and pelvic node irradiation (30 Gy over 3 weeks)
    b. All Stage IIA and some Stage IIB seminomas are treated with radiotherapy to the abdominal and pelvic lymph nodes: recurrence rates are 10% and 20% respectively
    c. Stage IIC disease treated by radiotherapy alone is associated with a 40% recurrence rate: chemotherapy is now becoming the initial treatment of choice in these patients with selected patients, including those with large nodal masses or a poor response to cytotoxics, having subsequent radiotherapy
    d. The inguinal nodes and scrotum are excluded from the treatment field unless a scrotal approach has been used, if the primary disease is locally advanced with invasion of the parietal tunica or if a previous orchidopexy or herniorrhaphy has been performed
    e. Localised radiotherapy may also be required in those patients with more advanced disease who receive chemotherapy and whose bulk disease does not respond adequately to the cytotoxic agents
3. Chemotherapy
    a. As Stage IIC seminomas show a high rate of recurrence if treated by radiotherapy alone, combination chemotherapy (bleomycin, etoposide and cisplatinum) is now the preferred treatment
    b. Combination chemotherapy is the treatment of choice in patients with disseminated disease (Stage III and IV)
    c. Patients who relapse after previous radiotherapy are also treated with combination chemotherapy

Treatment of teratoma
1. Orchidectomy
    a. Standard orchidectomy through an inguinal incision as described for seminoma is again indicated
    b. Surveillance at regular intervals for Stage 1 disease in patients whose elevated serum markers return to normal levels following orchidectomy is now becoming popular as only 10% of node negative patients will subsequently develop abdominal or pelvic lymph node metastases
    c. Patients are examined at monthly intervals in the first year, two monthly intervals in the second year and three monthly intervals in the third year
    d. Serum markers are measured at the same intervals

2. Radiotherapy
   a. Some centres continue to treat Stage I teratoma patients with the conventional adjuvant treatment of para-aortic and pelvic node irradiation (40 Gy over 4–5 weeks)
   b. Radiotherapy has no role in more advanced disease
3. Chemotherapy
   a. All teratomas of Stages II, III and IV are treated with combination chemotherapy
   b. Bleomycin, etoposide (VP 16) and cisplatinum is the currently favoured combination although other combinations which include vincristine and methotrexate are also used
   c. Patients treated in this way achieve a 75–90% clinical response rate depending on the volume of disease present
4. Retroperitoneal lymph node dissection
   a. In the USA para-aortic lymphadenectomy is used as a primary staging procedure to detect microscopic lymph node metastases: this is not common practice in the UK
   b. Post-chemotherapy resection of tumour masses is standard treatment for residual bulky disease; it is not only therapeutic but is also useful as a secondary staging procedure

Summary of treatment of germ cell tumours

Stage	Seminoma	Teratoma
I	Orchidectomy and surveillance ±Radiotherapy	Orchidectomy and surveillance ±Radiotherapy
IIA	Radiotherapy	Combination chemotherapy
IIB	Combination chemotherapy or Radiotherapy	Combination chemotherapy
IIC	Combination chemotherapy ±Radiotherapy to bulky disease	Combination chemotherapy
III	Combination chemotherapy ±Radiotherapy to bulky disease	Combination chemotherapy
IV	Combination chemotherapy ±Radiotherapy to bulky disease	Combination chemotherapy

Prognosis
The prognosis of testicular tumours is dependent on their stage at time of presentation, histological nature and degree of differentiation. The level and response to treatment of any

associated tumour markers are also important. Initial marker levels
correlate well with tumour bulk.

1. Type of tumour

Tumour	3-year survival (%)
Seminoma	85
Teratoma	50

2. Histological differentiation

Teratoma	3-year survival (%)
TD	92
MTI	52
MTU	38
MTT	19

3. Stage of disease

Seminoma	3-year survival (%)	5-year survival (%)
Stage I	97	95
Stage II	86	80
Stage III	70	65

FURTHER READING

Blandy J P, Oliver R T D 1984 Cancer of the testis. Br J Surg 71: 962–963
Blandy J P 1985 Role of surgery. J R Soc Med 78 Suppl 6: 32–34
Ellis M, Sikora K 1987 The current management of testicular cancer. Br J
    Urol 59: 2–9
Heyderman E 1985 Advances in pathology and immunocytochemistry. J R
    Soc Med 78 Suppl 6: 9–18
Hope-Stone H F 1985 Is radiotherapy defunct? J R Soc Med 78 Suppl
    6: 35–39
Husband J E 1985 Staging testicular tumours: the role of CT scanning. J R
    Soc Med 78 Suppl 6: 25–31
Light P A 1985 Tumour markers in testicular cancer. J R Soc Med 78 Suppl
    6: 19–24
Oliver R T D 1984 Testis cancer. Br J Hosp Med 31: 23–35
Peckham M J 1985 Orchidectomy for clinical Stage I testicular cancer:
    progress report of the Royal Marsden Hospital study. J R Soc Med 78
    Suppl 6: 41–42
Peckham M J, Hendry W F 1987 Testicular cancer. In: Hendry W F (ed)
    Recent Advances in Urology/Andrology. Churchill Livingstone, Edinburgh
    pp 279–312
Wilkinson P M 1985 Chemotherapy for non-seminomatous germ-cell
    tumours. J R Soc Med 78 Suppl 6: 43–47

PERCUTANEOUS NEPHROLITHOTOMY

Percutaneous renal surgery for the treatment of renal calculi avoids
the need for open surgery with its attendant morbidity and
mortality. Total hospital stay is reduced and patients are able to
return to their normal activities much sooner than after
conventional surgical procedures such as pyelolithotomy.

Technique

1. Percutaneous nephrolithotomy (PCNL) may be performed as a one- or two-stage procedure
2. Local anaesthesia usually requires supplementation with intra-venous benzodiazepines and narcotic analgesics; general anaesthesia is preferred for one-stage procedures
3. Antibiotic prophylaxis is given routinely
4. Renal collecting system is opacified by intra-venous or retrograde pyelography and a long thin needle inserted into the renal pelvis under fluoroscopic control
5. A wide-bore track is formed by passage of serial fascial dilators over a guide wire; a nephrostomy catheter is inserted to complete the first stage
6. Percutaneous endoscopy can be performed immediately but is more often carried out at the second stage after an interval of 5–7 days when the nephrostomy tube is removed and an Amplatz sheath inserted along its track; the nephroscope is passed through this sheath which protects the walls of the track
7. Rigid nephroscopes are used in preference to flexible fibre-optic instruments as they allow faster saline irrigation flow rates and the passage of larger instruments
8. Small stones (<1.5 cm in diameter) can be removed intact using stone-grasping forceps or a basket
9. Larger stones require fragmentation using ultrasonic (USL) or electro-hydraulic lithotripsy (EHL)
10. Following successful stone extraction the nephrostomy tube is replaced and left in situ for 48 hours; spontaneous healing of the nephrostomy track occurs after its final withdrawal

Indications

1. Calculi greater than 3 cm especially staghorn calculi
2. Impacted upper ureteric stone
3. After extra-corporeal shock wave lithotripsy if there are residual calculi and especially if they cause ureteric obstruction
4. As an emergency procedure in acute hydronephrosis, pyonephrosis and obstructive renal failure

Contraindications

1. Coagulation disorders
2. Pregnancy

Complications

1. Pyelo-venous reflux of irrigating fluid
2. Ureteric obstruction by stone fragments or blood clot
3. Perforation of renal pelvis
4. Haemorrhage
5. Arterio-venous fistula
6. Bacteraemia and septicaemia

FURTHER READING

Miller R A 1986 A review of the new methods for the treatment of renal and
   ureteric calculi. In: Russell R C G (ed) Recent Advances in Surgery Vol 12.
   Churchill Livingstone, Edinburgh pp 215–230
Webb D R, Payne S R, Wickham J E A 1986 Extracorporeal shockwave
   lithotripsy and percutaneous renal surgery: comparisons, combinations
   and conclusions. Br J Urol 58: 1–5

EXTRA-CORPOREAL SHOCK WAVE LITHOTRIPSY

Extra-corporeal shock wave lithotripsy (ESWL) is a completely non-
invasive method of disintegrating urinary calculi. The discomfort
associated with conventional surgical treatment is avoided and the
length of hospital stay greatly reduced. Successful fragmentation of
large calculi is followed by the natural passage of smaller stone
fragments.

Technique
1. Either epidural or general anaesthesia is used
2. Patient is placed in water bath at 37°C and positioned over an
   elliptical electro-hydraulic shock wave generator
3. Electrical explosion in the generator produces a shock wave
   which is accurately focussed onto the calculus with the aid of
   two dimensional fluoroscopic screening and a computer
4. Individual shock waves are synchronised with the patient's
   electrocardiogram which is continuously monitored
5. 500–1500 individual shocks given over 30–60 minutes are
   required to fragment the calculus depending on its size
6. Diuresis is obtained by a high oral fluid intake for 48 hours and
   is required to eliminate the stone fragments, which have an
   average diameter of 2 mm

Indications
1. Radio-opaque renal calculi <3 cm in diameter
2. Ureteric calculi above the iliac crest

Contraindications
1. Pregnancy
2. Distal ureteric obstruction
3. Impacted ureteric stone
4. Calculi >3 cm in diameter
5. Obesity (body weight >120 kg)
6. Severe cardio-pulmonary disease
7. Cardiac pacemaker
8. Haemorrhagic diathesis

Complications
1. Hypotension
2. Cardiac arrhythmias
3. Ureteric obstruction

FURTHER READING

Miller R A 1986 A review of the new methods for the treatment of renal and ureteric calculi. In: Russell R C G (ed) Recent Advances in Surgery vol 12. Churchill Livingstone, Edinburgh, pp 215–230

Webb D R, Payne S R, Wickham J E A 1986 Extracorporeal shockwave lithotripsy and percutaneous renal surgery. Br J Urol 58: 1–5

Breast cancer

BREAST CANCER: STAGING, DIAGNOSIS AND SCREENING

Introduction

Breast carcinoma is a major cause of death in middle-aged and elderly women in the Western world. The incidence of breast cancer is slowly increasing and one in twenty women can expect to develop the disease within a lifetime. The mortality has changed little over the last 50 years about half of all women still dieing within 5 years of diagnosis.

Staging: TNM classification

T: Primary tumour
TO   No evidence of primary tumour
TIS   Carcinoma in situ
T1   Tumour <2 cm diameter without fixation
T2   Tumour 2–5 cm diameter without fixation
T3   Tumour >5 cm diameter
T4   Direct extension of a tumour of any size to the overlying skin or chest wall
N: Regional lymph node metastases
N0   No palpable lymph nodes
N1   Mobile ipsilateral axillary lymph nodes
N2   Fixed ipsilateral axillary lymph nodes
N3   Ipsilateral infra-clavicular or supra-clavicular lymph nodes
M: Distant metastases
M0   No evidence of distant metastases
M1   Distant metastases present

Diagnosis

Diagnosis of breast cancer based solely on clinical examination is notoriously unreliable. Pre-operative diagnostic accuracy can be improved by mammography, ultrasonography, aspiration cytology or needle or drill biopsy. An accurate pre-operative diagnosis allows planning of definitive treatment and proper counselling of the patient.

1. Mammography
   a. The incidence of false-negative and false-positive results may be as high as 10–20% but these figures should fall with improved radiological techniques and increased expertise in interpreting mammogram films
   b. Mammographic features suggesting the presence of a malignant breast tumour include:
      (i) poorly circumscribed lesion of increased tissue density with irregular margins often with a stellate appearance
      (ii) infiltration of surrounding tissues with retraction of trabeculae and increased vascularity
      (iii) localised spiculated microcalcification of variable density
      (iv) lymph nodes may be visible in the axilla
   c. In contrast the mammographic appearances of benign breast disease are:
      (i) well-circumscribed lesions of uniform density
      (ii) calcification which is not clustered and may be throughout the breast often within blood vessels or the skin
2. Ultrasonography
   a. In expert hands static B mode ultrasound mammography is more sensitive than conventional X-ray mammography in the pre-operative diagnosis of breast carcinoma
   b. Satisfactory imaging of the radiologically dense breast is difficult with X-ray mammography but is usually possible with ultrasound
   c. Ultrasound localisation may also improve the sensivity of fine needle aspiration cytology
3. Aspiration cytology
   a. Fine needle aspiration cytology (FNAC) is easily performed without local anaesthesia in the outpatient department but an experienced cytologist is essential
   b. Epithelial cells from a breast carcinoma can be examined within a few minutes of aspiration and a diagnosis of malignancy can usually be confirmed
   c. False-positive reporting is extremely rare
   d. Differentiation between carcinoma in situ and invasive carcinoma is not possible
   e. Epithelial cells are occasionally not obtained either because of a poor sampling technique or in very fibrous tumours where the proportion of epithelial cells is very low
   f. With good aspirates the incidence of false negative reporting is low and may be caused by unrepresentative sampling
4. Histological examination of biopsy material
   a. Histopathological examination should always be used to confirm a diagnosis of breast carcinoma

b. A pre-operative histological diagnosis of breast cancer can be determined from material obtained by Tru-cut needle or drill biopsy
c. Both techniques can be performed under local anaesthesia
d. False-positive results are extremely rare
e. Distinction between invasive and in situ carcinoma is possible
f. If an adequate pre-operative diagnosis has not been made either an incisional or excisional surgical biopsy can be used to provide material for frozen section histological examination

Screening for early cancer

1. Clinical examination
   a. Palpation of the breasts by a trained observer or self-examination produces a small but significant reduction in the size of operable breast tumours at presentation in women aged between 45 and 65 years
   b. No significant difference in the degree of lymph node involvement has so far been shown
   c. To date no improvement in survival can be ascribed to breast self-examination and this is therefore not an effective screening method when used alone
2. Mammography
   a. Mammographic screening to detect impalpable breast carcinomas has been shown to reduce the incidence of Stage II disease by 25% and deaths from breast carcinoma by up to 30% in women aged 50–65 years
   b. The incidence of detecting breast cancer in screened patients of this age is 4 per 1000 at prevalence screening and 1 per 1000 at subsequent incidence screening
   c. Routine mammographic screening is not normally performed in women under 40 years of age as the incidence of asymptomatic breast cancer is too low to justify its use
   d. A single lateral oblique view mammogram of high quality is sufficient in most cases; this reduces both the cost of the examination and the radiation exposure
   e. The ideal frequency of further examinations has yet to be determined but a 3-year interval between screening mammography is probably safe
   f. Successful biopsy of impalpable breast lesions detected by screening mammography may require mammographic localisation procedures: a skilled team including a surgeon, radiologist and pathologist is essential
   g. In the presence of a palpable breast tumour which can be confirmed as a carcinoma by aspiration cytology mammography may be used to detect a synchronous non-palpable tumour in the ipsilateral or contralateral breast

High-risk groups

Risk factors recognised for the development of breast cancer
include the following:

1. Age > 45 years
2. Carcinoma of contralateral breast
3. Family history of breast cancer in first degree relatives
4. Nulliparity
5. First full-term pregnancy after 30 years of age
6. Early menarche and late natural menopause
7. Early artificial menopause
8. Previous fibrocystic disease especially in those cases with
   proliferative epithelial changes particularly if cellular atypia is
   present
9. High levels of dietary fat

Prognostic indices

1. Size of primary tumour
2. Lymph node status
3. Histopathological (Bloom and Richardson) grade
4. Oestrogen receptor (ER) status
5. Metastatic spread
6. Menopausal status

FURTHER READING

Coombes R C, Powles T J, Abbott M et al 1980 Physical tests for distant
    metastases in patients with breast cancer. J R Soc Med 73: 617–623
Dowle C S, Mitchell A, Elston C W et al 1987 Preliminary results of the
    Nottingham breast self-examination education programme. Br J Surg
    74: 217–219
Ellman R 1987 Breast cancer screening. J R Soc Med 80: 665–666
Frank H A, Hall F M, Steer M L 1976 Preoperative localisation of nonpalpable
    breast lesions demonstrated by mammography. N Eng J Med
    295: 259–260
Knox R A, Marshall T, Kingston R D 1984 Fine needle aspiration breast
    cytology in district general hospital practice. Clin Oncol 10: 369–373
Mansi J L, Berger U, Easton D et al 1987 Micrometastases in bone marrow
    in patients with primary breast cancer: evaluation as an early predictor of
    bone metastases. Br Med J 295: 1093–1096
Tabar L, Gad A, Holmberg L H et al 1985 Reduction in mortality from breast
    cancer after mass screening with mammography. Lancet i: 829–832
Tate J J T, Royle G T, McDonald P, Guyer P B, Taylor I 1987 X-ray and
    ultrasound localisation of non-palpable breast lesions and difficulties in
    management. J R Soc Med 80: 678–680
Verbeek A L M, Hendricks J H C L, Holland R et al 1984 Reduction in breast
    cancer mortality through mass screening with modern mammography.
    Lancet i: 1222–1224
Warwick D J, Smallwood J A, Guyer P B, Dewbury K C, Taylor I 1988
    Ultrasound mamography in the management of breast cancer. Br J Surg
    75: 243–245

Williams C M, Dickerson J W T 1987 Dietary fat, hormones and breast
    cancer: the cell membrane as a possible site of interaction of these two
    risk factors. Eur J Surg Oncol 13: 89–104

TREATMENT OF 'EARLY' BREAST CANCER

Definition
An early breast carcinoma is one in which there is no clinical
evidence of growth or dissemination beyond T2, N1.

Detection of occult metastases
Many patients with 'early' breast cancer will eventually die of
metastatic disease but at the time of presentation these occult
distant metastases are usually impossible to demonstrate because
of the low resolution of the investigative techniques available.
Routine screening for metastases by use of the following
techniques is usually reserved for patients with palpable nodal
disease:
1. Chest radiography
2. Radiographic skeletal survey
3. Isotope bone scintigraphy
4. Ultrasonographic liver scan
5. Radio-isotope liver scan
In patients with Stage I disease the yield of true positive scans is
less than 2%.

Surgical treatment
Provided local surgical excision is accompanied by adequate local
radiotherapy the nature of the primary surgical treatment of breast
carcinoma has no effect on the development of distant metastases
or the patient's long term survival. The main aims of surgical
treatment are therefore to prevent local recurrence and to minimise
functional disability, cosmetic defects and psychological morbidity.
1. Wide local excision of tumour (tumourectomy, lumpectomy)
    a. Without radical local radiotherapy this technique produces
       unacceptably poor results, more than a third of patients
       developing local tumour recurrence within three years
    b. The tumour should be excised with a 1 cm margin of
       surrounding normal breast tissue and the excision margins
       should be free of tumour when subsequently examined
       histologically
    c. Controversy exists about the staging and treatment of the
       axilla following local excision of a breast carcinoma
    d. Some surgeons stage the axilla by sampling up to four
       axillary nodes and then irradiate the axilla
    e. Other surgeons perform a radical axillary node dissection
       and then exclude the axilla from subsequent radiotherapy
       fields

    f. Major prospective randomised clinical trials have confirmed that conservative surgery when combined with radiotherapy produces results equivalent to those obtained by mastectomy

    g. Women with large primary breast tumours or multifocal disease are not suitable for conservative surgery

2. Simple mastectomy
   a. The entire breast is excised having first obtained histological confirmation of the clinical diagnosis
   b. None of the underlying muscles are removed or divided and only the lower axillary contents are biopsied

3. Modified radical (Patey) mastectomy
   a. Pectoralis major muscle is preserved but the insertion of pectoralis minor is detached from the coracoid process to allow easier access to the axilla
   b. Less cosmetic disturbance is produced than in the classical radical mastectomy but a similar axillary lymph node dissection is possible

4. Radical (Halsted) mastectomy
   a. Apart from the sternal head of pectoralis major which is preserved both pectoral muscles are removed thus facilitating access to the axillary contents which are cleared more easily than in the Patey dissection
   b. Loss of the pectoralis major muscle produces a marked cosmetic defect

5. Extended radical (Urban) mastectomy
   a. The Halsted mastectomy is extended to include excision of the internal thoracic (mammary) lymph nodes
   b. Post-operative morbidity and mortality are both very high

6. Reconstructive surgery
   a. Patients requiring mastectomy can be offered reconstructive surgery either at the time of mastectomy or at a later date
   b. Breast reconstruction can be performed using prosthetic implants, including tissue expanders, or myocutaneous flaps, the latissimus dorsi flap being most popular at present

Radiotherapy

1. Breast
   a. Following local excision of a breast carcinoma radical radiotherapy is required to prevent recurrence of the tumour in the residual breast tissue
   b. Megavoltage external beam radiotherapy begins 10–14 days following tumour excision and is given as daily fractions; fractionation and duration of treatment vary from one unit to another
   c. A boost to the site of the primary tumour is usually provided by an external beam or less commonly by ^{192}Ir wire implants inserted under general anaesthetic

    d. Local skin changes including erythema, desquamation and pigmentation accompany the radiotherapy but resolve spontaneously

    e. Long-term complications are uncommon and include telangiectasia and fibrosis but the overall functional and cosmetic results are reported as satisfactory, good or excellent in over 80% of patients

2. Regional lymph nodes

    a. Unless complete axillary node clearance has been performed external beam radiotherapy to the axilla is usually standard practice for tumours in the lateral half of the breast

    b. A 10 Gy boost to the axilla may be given if axillary lymph node biopsy has revealed tumour deposits

    c. Standard treatment involves a separate anterior field to the supra-clavicular fossa

    d. The internal mammary chain is usually treated especially in medially situated tumours

Adjuvant cytotoxic chemotherapy

Given that many patients die of metastatic disease regardless of the form of local therapy used to treat their primary tumour attention has been focussed on the treatment of possible micrometastases at the time of initial presentation. A number of trials to determine the possible benefits of adjuvant chemotherapy at the time of surgical treatment of primary breast cancer have now been reported.

1. The National Surgical Adjuvant Breast Project (NSABP) L-phenylalanine mustard (melphalan) trial showed a reduction in mortality of 25% after a 10-year follow-up in patients less than 50 years old compared with controls

2. The Milan Cancer Institute trial which used a combination adjuvant regimem consisting of cyclophosphamide, methotrexate and 5-fluorouracil (CMF) showed a similar reduction in mortality in pre-menopausal patients

3. Most other trials have confirmed the benefit of adjuvant cytotoxic chemotherapy in pre-menopausal patients with involved axillary lymph nodes and indicated that the survival benefit is greatest when less than four axillary nodes are involved by tumour

4. Post-menopausal patients derive no benefit

5. Initial studies evaluated regimens lasting 2 years; a 6-month course is probably as effective

6. Beneficial effect of adjuvant therapy may be related to suppression of ovarian function

7. Adjuvant therapy produces several toxic side effects and many surgeons feel that the morbidity associated with the treatment does not justify the increased survival which might be obtained

Adjuvant endocrine therapy
1. Ovarian ablation
   a. In pre-menopausal and peri-menopausal patients with small tumours ovarian ablation has produced an increase in both disease-free survival and overall survival in several studies
   b. May be performed by surgical oophorectomy or ovarian irradiation (radiation menopause)
2. Tamoxifen
   a. The relatively non-toxic anti-oestrogen agent tamoxifen (Nolvadex) competes with oestradiol for a cytoplasmic oestrogen receptor which controls DNA transcription
   b. It may also have a direct cytocidal effect which is independent of oestrogen receptor status
   c. In a controlled trial of adjuvant tamoxifen disease-free survival was increased by up to 25% and total survival was prolonged by 15% in post-menopausal patients receiving adjuvant tamoxifen, 20 mg daily for 2 years, following surgery and local radiotherapy
   d. The optimum duration of adjuvant tamoxifen treatment is not yet determined
   e. Tamoxifen is usually tolerated well and as yet long-term therapy does not appear to have any serious side effects

Management of ductal carcinoma in situ (DCIS)
1. Ductal carcinoma in situ (DCIS) is observed in less than 2% of all cases of symptomatic breast cancer but in up to 20% of those tumours which are detected by mammographic screening
2. Microcalcification is a characteristic feature of DCIS and one that is readily detected by mammography
3. DCIS is frequently multicentric but lesions do not tend to occur in the opposite breast
4. Simple mastectomy will cure all patients with DCIS and until recently has been the standard method of treatment
5. Axillary node dissection is not required as no nodal metastases will be present provided microinvasion has not occurred
6. Mastectomy is still recommended in cases of diffuse changes indicating multiple foci of DCIS throughout the breast
7. Where only a localised focus of DCIS is present local excision with careful clinical and mammographic surveillance is possible
8. In all cases treated conservatively surveillance must be scrupulous as up to 30% of patients may subsequently develop an invasive carcinoma in the ipsilateral breast

Management of lobular carcinoma in situ (LCIS)
1. Lobular carcinoma in situ (LCIS) is rarely detected by mammography and is usually an incidental finding on biopsy of an otherwise benign palpable breast lesion

2. 15–35% of patients with LCIS treated by biopsy alone will subsequently develop an invasive breast carcinoma
3. The risk of developing an invasive breast carcinoma in the contralateral breast is similar to that of the breast in which the LCIS is first detected
4. Prophylactic bilateral mastectomy has been advocated in the past
5. Many surgeons now perform local excision and arrange regular clinical and mamographic surveillance

FURTHER READING

Anderson J, Blichert-Toft M, Dyreborg U 1987 In situ carcinomas of the breast. Types, growth pattern, diagnosis and treatment. Eur J Surg Oncol 13: 105–111

Ashford R F U, Phillips R H, Coe M A 1984 Conservative excision and radiotherapy for early breast cancer – an acceptable alternative. Clin Oncol 10: 45–58

Berstock D A, Baum M 1982 Adjuvant therapy for early breast cancer. Hosp Update 8: 1277–1284

Bluming A Z, Dosik G, Lowitz B et al 1986 Treatment of primary breast cancer without mastectomy. Ann Surg 204: 136–147

Bonnadonna G, Valgussa P 1987 Current status of adjuvant chemotherapy for breast cancer. Seminars in Oncology 14: 8–22

Bulman A S, Cassoni A M, Ellis H 1985 The functional results following primary treatment of breast cancer with conservation. Eur J Surg Oncol 11: 247–249

Chetty U, Forrest A P M 1986 Breast conservation Br J Surg 73: 599–600

Cooke T 1987 Adjuvant systemic therapy for carcinoma of the breast. In: Taylor I (ed) Progress in Surgery Vol 2. Churchill Livingstone, Edinburgh pp 188–197

Fisher B, Bauer M, Margolese R et al 1985 Five-year results of a randomized clinical trial comparing total mastectomy and segmental mastectomy with or without radiation in the treatment of breast cancer. N Eng J Med 312: 665–673

Henderson I C 1988 Adjuvant therapy for breast cancer. New Eng J Med 318: 443–444

Hughes L E, Webster D J T 1980 The treatment of early breast cancer. Br J Hosp Med 23: 22–31

Nolvadex Adjuvant Trial Organisation 1985 Controlled trial of tamoxifen as single adjuvant agent in management of early breast cancer. Lancet i: 836–840

Padmanabhan N, Howell A, Rubens R D 1986 Mechanism of action of adjuvant chemotherapy in early breast cancer. Lancet ii: 413–414

Pritchard K I 1987 Current status of adjuvant endocrine therapy for resectable breast cancer. Seminars in Oncology 14: 23–33

Riberio G, Palmer M K 1983 Adjuvant tamoxifen for operable carcinoma of the breast: report of clinical trial by the Christie Hospital and Holt Radium Institute. Br Med J 286: 827–830

van Dongen J A, Bartelink H, Fentiman I S, Peterse J L 1987 Ductal carcinoma in situ (DCIS) of the breast–a therapeutic dilemma. Eur J Surg Oncol 13: 123–125

Wilson A J, Baum M, Brinkley D M 1985 Six year results of a controlled trial of tamoxifen as single adjuvant agent in management of early breast cancer. World J Surg 9: 756–774

TREATMENT OF ADVANCED BREAST CANCER

Definition
1. Breast tumours staged beyond T2, N1 at the time of presentation
2. Loco-regional recurrent breast carcinoma
3. Presence of distant metastatic disease (M1)

General guidelines
1. In most centres simple hormonal treatment is the first line of treatment in patients with metastatic breast cancer
2. Cytotoxic chemotherapy is used in those patients who fail to respond to endocrine manipulation and those who subsequently relapse
3. Radiotherapy is used in previously unirradiated patients to treat locally advanced primary disease or locally recurrent breast cancer
4. Radiotherapy and surgery may be required for the treatment of specific complications arising from localised metastatic disease

Simple hormonal manipulation
In pre-menopausal patients the first line of treatment is tamoxifen. Oophorectomy may be considered in those patients who show an objective response. With subsequent relapse treatment with aminoglutethimide should be considered. Progestogens and androgens may also be useful.

Post-menopausal patients are initially treated with tamoxifen. Further endocrine therapy would comprise aminogluthemide, androgens or oestrogens.

In all cases knowledge of the current receptor status will help select the most appropriate treatment and predict the response to it.
1. Tamoxifen
   a. The synthetic anti-oestrogen tamoxifen (Nolvadex), given orally in a dose of 20–40 mg daily, is now the most widely used hormonal treatment in advanced breast cancer
   b. Overall response rate is between 25% and 55% and is dependent on menopausal status
   c. Response rate correlates well with oestrogen receptor (ER) status
   d. Response to tamoxifen accurately predicts response to subsequent oophorectomy

    e. Most side effects are mild and include hot flushes, menstrual disturbances, fluid retention, anorexia, nausea and vomiting

    f. Transient thrombocytopenia and leucopenia are also seen and tamoxifen may cause a temporary flare with hypercalcaemia

2. Oophorectomy

    a. Ovarian ablation may be performed surgically or by external beam radiotherapy (radiation menopause)

    b. Indicated in pre-menopausal and early post-menopausal women

    c. Overall response rates of up to 30% are usually achieved with an average duration of response of 12 months

    d. Patients with oestrogen-receptor positive (ER-positive) tumours may show response rates greater than 50% whereas remission is achieved in less than 10% of those with ER-negative tumours

3. Aminoglutethimide

    a. Aminoglutethimide (Orimetin) inhibits adrenal steroid production and the conversion of androgens to oestrogens in peripheral tissues

    b. Adequate glucocorticoid replacement therapy must be given for the duration of treatment

    c. In general the 'medical adrenalectomy' produced by aminoglutethimide is as effective as a surgical adrenalectomy

    d. Indicated in post-menopausal patients or those who have been previously treated by oophorectomy

    e. Patients who have previously shown a good response to simple endocrine ablation and those with predominantly skeletal metastases are most likely to have an objective response

    f. Side effects include a transitory maculo-papular rash, and a characteristic syndrome of somnolence, lethargy nausea and dizziness

4. Progestogens

    a. Progestational agents may be as effective as oestrogens but have fewer side effects

    b. Examples include megestrol acetate (Megace) and medroxyprogesterone acetate (Provera)

    c. Two months continuous therapy may be required to produce a measureable response

    d. Response rates of 30–40% are usually obtained

    e. When progestogens are used as a second line therapy after tamoxifen a 30% response rate can still be expected

5. Androgen therapy

    a. Various androgens are still used to a limited extent as second and third line hormonal therapy in metastatic breast carcinoma

   b. Examples include nandrolone decanoate (Deca-Durabolin) and drostanolone propionate (Masteril)
   c. Masculinising effects are inevitable and in general androgens are associated with a lower response rate than oestrogens
6 Cortico-steroid therapy
   a. Cortico-steroids such as prednisolone and dexamethasone produce a response rate of about 25% which is independent of age or menopausal status
   b. Steroids induce a feeling of well-being and are particularly useful in the treatment of painful skeletal metastases and cerebral metastases
   c. Important in the control of malignant hypercalcaemia
7. Oestrogen therapy
   a. Diethylstilboestrol 5 mg 8-hourly is used as second-line therapy in post-menopausal patients
   b. Objective response is produced in 25–40% of all post-menopausal patients
   c. Response correlates well with oestrogen receptor status being over 50% in patients with ER-positive tumours and less than 10% in those with ER-negative tumours
   d. Side effects include nausea and vomiting, fluid retention and vaginal discharge; tumour flares with hypercalcaemia may also occur
   e. Ethinyloestradiol 1 mg 8-hourly is probably as effective as diethylstilboestrol but has fewer side effects
   f. A further remission on cessation of oestrogen therapy can be expected in one third of patients who showed an initial response and later progressed

Major endocrine ablation
Increased availability of various methods of hormonal manipulation and improved cytotoxic regimes have led to a decline in the number of major endocrine ablations that are now performed. Very few patients are now selected for this form of treatment which should only be undertaken in patients who show an objective response to simpler forms of hormonal manipulation.
  1. Bilateral adrenalectomy
     a. A major surgical procedure which should only be undertaken if simple endocrine manipulation has previously been performed and shown to be effective
     b. Replacement steroid therapy is required and the patient is susceptible to Addisonian crises
     c. Response can be expected in 25% of cases with an average remission in successful responders of 18 months being achieved

2. Hypophysectomy
    a. Hypophysectomy usually provides better response rates than adrenalectomy a successful response being achieved in just over one third of patients
    b. Average length of remission achieved is 3 years
    c. Patient management is easier as aldosterone and catecholamine production is not disturbed
    d. Diabeters insipidus requires treatment with vasopressin; argipressin (Pitressin) is given by subcutaneous or intra-muscular injection, lypressin (Syntopressin) by intra-nasal spray
    e. Hypophysectomy may be performed surgically via the trans-cranial (frontal) route but this is a major neurosurgical procedure associated with significant morbidity and mortality; it is unsuitable as a routine procedure
    f. The trans-ethmoidal, trans-sphenoidal route is an alternative which is generally safer although meningitis may occur and persistent CSF rhinorrhoea is an important complication
    g. Radioactive yttrium implants often produce incomplete pituitary ablation but the procedure is relatively minor and easily repeated; complications include radiation damage to the adjacent optic chiasma with visual field defects and meningitis with CSF rhinorrhoea

Factors predicting a favourable response to hormonal manipulation
1. Long disease-free interval
2. Good response to previous hormonal manipulation
3. Late post-menopausal status
4. ER-positive tumours
5. Advanced local disease without visceral metastases

Cytotoxic chemotherapy
1. Single agent chemotherapy
    a. Doxorubicin (Adriamycin) is the most effective single chemotherapeutic agent in breast cancer
    b. A 40% response rate can be expected when it is used as a first line cytotoxic agent
    c. A cumulative dose of 450–550 mg/m^2 should not be exceeded if the risk of cardiac failure is to be avoided
2. Cyclical combination chemotherapy
    a. Generally achieves a higher response rate than use of single cytotoxic agents
    b. A commonly used combination is cyclophosphamide, methotrexate, 5-fluorouracil, vincristine and predinsolone (CMFVP)

    c. A four-weekly cycle of chemotherapy allows time for bone marrow stem-cell recovery and minimises the toxic effects of the cytotoxic agents

    d. Overall response rates of 50–80% can be expected with 15–20% of patients showing a complete response

    e. Despite an initial favourable response to chemotherapy the median survival of patients with metastatic breast carcinoma is prolonged by only a few months

    f. Combination chemotherapy with mitoxantrone (Novantrone), methotrexate and mitomycin-C has recently been shown to give a response rate of 60% but has fewer side effects than conventional cytotoxic regimens

3. Intra-cavity chemotherapy

    a. Aspiration of pleural effusions provides symptomatic relief of dyspnoea; instillation of an alkylating agent such as triethylenethiophosporamide (Thiotepa) is used to prevent recurrence

    b. Similarly abdominal paracentesis and intra-cavity cytotoxics are used in cases of malignant ascites

    c. More recently inactivated Corynebacterium parvum organisms (Coparvax) have been instilled into the pleural or peritoneal cavities to treat malignant effusions

Factors predicting a favourable response to cytotoxic chemotherapy

1. Small tumour burden
2. Good performance status
3. Absence of visceral metastases

Radiotherapy
Radiotherapy is indicated in the following situations:
1. Locally advanced primary breast carcinoma
2. Localised skin and lymph node metastases
3. Painful localised skeletal metastases
4. Superior mediastinal obstruction
5. Spinal cord compression
6. Following internal fixation of pathological long bone fractures

Surgical treatment
1. Laminectomy for spinal cord compression by metastatic deposits
2. Ureteric catheterisation for obstructive uropathy
3. Internal fixation of pathological fractures of long bones
4. Prophylactic internal fixation of skeletal metastases

Treatment of malignant hypercalcaemia
Up to 30% of patients with skeletal metastases due to breast cancer will develop hypercalcaemia which may be precipitated by

hormonal therapy especially tamoxifen. Hypercalcaemia in advanced breast cancer is associated with a poor prognosis. It should be suspected in the following situations:

1. Deterioration in general condition
2. Severe increase in bone pain
3. Anorexia, nausea and vomiting
4. Progressive weakness and lethargy
5. Oliguric renal failure
6. Coma

Having diagnosed malignant hypercalcaemia the following therapeutic manoeuvres should be undertaken:

1. Discontinue any recently commenced hormone therapy
2. Intra-venous saline
   a. Dehydration is corrected, the effective intra-vascular volume restored and diuresis promoted
   b. With a marked saline diuresis increased calcium excretion is achieved
   c. Increased saline and calcium excretion can be maintained by treatment with frusemide
   d. Hypokalaemia should be prevented by adequate replacement therapy
3. Inorganic phosphate
   a. Either oral or intra-venous phosphate is given the latter having a more rapid effect
   b. Hypocalcaemia with tetany and extra-skeletal calcification may complicate phosphate therapy
4. Cortico-steroids
   a. Large doses of prednisolone 60–80 mg per day are given
   b. Reduction in serum calcium is relatively slow often taking 5–10 days to achieve a maximal effect
5. Mithramycin
   a. A cytotoxic antibiotic which prevents osteoclastic function by inhibiting RNA synthesis
   b. Produces a fall in serum calcium level within 6 hours
   c. Side effects include thrombocytopaenia, hepatitis and renal failure
6. Calcitonin
   a. This peptide hormone produces a fall in serum calcium within 2–4 hours
   b. Apart from occasional allergic reactions side effects are uncommon

FURTHER READING

Davis H L 1983 Management of hypercalcaemia in cancer. Reviews on Endocrine-related cancer 15: 15–22

Vascular surgery

VASCULAR GRAFTS

Indications for use of vascular grafts
1. Tissue ischaemia
   a. Acute, e.g. trauma, thrombosis
   b. Chronic, e.g. occlusive vascular disease
2. Arterial replacement
   a. Aneurysm repair
   b. En-bloc tumour excision
3. Venous replacement
   a. Trauma
   b. Elective reconstruction for valve insufficiency or following en-bloc tumour excision
4. Vascular access, e.g. haemodialysis

General principles for the use of arterial bypass grafts
1. Ensure good inflow to graft by excluding or correcting proximal disease
2. Ensure good run-off from the graft; arterial bypass is contraindicated in the presence of severe distal disease
3. Avoid kinking or compression of graft
4. Avoid narrowing graft at anastomoses
5. Prevent intimal dissections by careful technique; intimal flaps may need to be anchored by fine axial sutures

Requirements for an ideal arterial graft
1. Non-thrombogenic flow surface
2. Resistant to infection and biodegradation
3. Predictable host tissue response
4. Elastic properties similar to those of host artery
5. Available in a wide range of lengths and diameters
6. Ease of storage with long shelf life
7. Minimum preparation prior to use
8. Ease of handling and suturing

Biological grafts

1. Reversed autogenous long saphenous vein graft
   a. Easily accessible and inexpensive but harvesting may be time consuming
   b. The graft of choice for femoro-popliteal and coronary artery bypass procedures
   c. External diameter should exceed 4 mm
   d. During harvesting the vein must be handled gently and kept moist
   e. The patency of femoro-popliteal bypass grafts is related to the indication for the graft, its length and the quality of the run off

Patency of reversed autogenous saphenous vein femoro-popliteal bypass grafts (%)

	5 years	10 years
Indication:		
Intermittent claudication	75	45
Rest pain	40	20
Distal run off:		
Good	70	40
Poor	40	30
Length of graft:		
Short (above-knee)	80	40
Long (below-knee)	30	25

2. In situ long saphenous vein graft
   a. Valves are destroyed using special valve strippers, valvulotomes or micro-scissors inserted through transverse venotomies
   b. All tributaries are ligated to prevent development of arterio-venous fistulae
   c. Vasa vasorum of the vein remain intact and hence its nutrition is preserved
   d. The graft of choice for femoro-distal bypass procedures
   e. As the graft narrows distally blood flow increases and is maximal at the distal anastomosis thus tending to maintain its patency
   f. Multiple anastomoses to the distal calf arteries using tributaries of the saphenous vein are often feasible
   g. Saphenous vein with a diameter of only 2.5–3 mm may be used
   h. Provided cases are well selected an 80% 1 year patency rate for femoro-tibial bypass procedures is obtainable
3. Allografts, e.g. human umbilical cord vein allograft (HUCVAG)
   a. Lined by intima and has no branches or valves

  b. Available in large quantities but usually in limited lengths; a longer graft can be made by joining two or more grafts by end-to-end anastomisis
  c. Chemical processing involves tanning with glutaraldehyde which renders the graft non-antigenic and increases its tensile strength
  d. Dardik biograft is strengthened by an outer polyester mesh wrap to prevent aneurysmal dilatation
  e. Used for below knee femoro-popliteal and femoro-distal bypasses when saphenous vein is not available
4. Heterografts, e.g. bovine carotid arterial grafts
  a. Prepared by digestion of bovine carotid artery in protease enzymes then tanned with dialdehyde starch or glutaraldehyde to produce a tube of non-antigenic collagen
  b. High incidence of calcification and aneurysmal dilatation when used for arterial bypass but still used for vascular access

Synthetic grafts
1. Dacron
    A synthetic fibre made from the polymerisation of polyethylene terephthalate
  a. Woven dacron
      (i) Fibres are packed tightly together to produce a material with low porosity
      (ii) Only slight haemorrhage through graft wall occurs following implantation and preclotting is not essential
      (iii) Minimal ingrowth by fibrous tissue
      (iv) Prosthetic material of choice for repair of ruptured abdominal aortic aneurysms
  b. Knitted dacron
      (i) High porosity allows penetration by granulation tissue and formation of endothelium
      (ii) Marked leakage of blood through the graft wall occurs after implantation and therefore it should be preclotted before use
      (iii) Easier to handle, more conformable and less likely to fray than woven dacron
      (iv) Suitable for replacement or bypass of the aorta and the visceral and proximal limb arteries
  c. Dacron velour
      (i) Highly porous graft which must always be preclotted prior to use
      (ii) Should not be used in the presence of coagulation defects
      (iii) Internal velour promotes formation of pseudointima and endothelium
      (iv) External velour encourages adherence of fibrous tissues

2. Expanded polytetrafluorethylene (PTFE), e.g. Gore-Tex,
   Impragraft
   a. Hydrophobic polymer with a high electro-negative surface
      charge
   b. PTFE is a microporous, non-elastic strong material
   c. Inert smooth surface prevents platelet deposition giving a
      low thrombogenic potential
   d. PTFE allows tissue ingrowth and neointima formation
   e. Preclotting is not required
   f. Gore-Tex grafts are reinforced by a thin outer layer of high
      tensile strength PTFE to reduce the possibility of aneurysm
      formation
   g. Used for above-knee and below-knee femoro-popliteal and
      extra-anatomic bypasses eg axillo-femoral and femoro-
      femoral bypasses
   h. Haemorrhage from suture holes at the anastomoses may
      prove difficult especially in patients with coagulation defects
   i. Pseudoaneursym formation at puncture sites limits its use
      for vascular access
   j. As with autogenous vein patency is related to the length of
      the graft, the symptoms present and the quality of the distal
      run-off

Patency of expanded PTFE femoro-popliteal bypass grafts (%)

	1 year	3 years	5 years
Length of graft:			
Short (above-knee)	80	75	65
Long (below-knee)	55	45	25
Symptoms:			
Intermittent claudication	85	75	65
Rest pain	75	60	35

Complications of synthetic arterial grafts
1. Haemorrhage
   a. Haemorrhage through the graft wall is a potential problem
      with all synthetic grafts especially those of high porosity
   b. It can be minimised by adequate preclotting of the graft
      before systemic heparinisation
2. Infection
   a. Graft sepsis is associated with a high mortality and
      morbidity, the rate of amputation being greatly increased
   b. Manifestations include fever, purulent wound discharge,
      false aneurysm formation, septic infarcts and septicaemia
   c. Infection of an abdominal aortic graft may lead to aorto-
      enteric fistulation presenting with gastro-intestinal
      haemorrhage and associated with a high mortality

    d. Graft infections are often caused by a mixed growth of organisms: Staphylococci usually infect grafts placed in the inguinal region; coliform and other aerobic Gram-negative organisms are often cultured from infected aorto-iliac grafts

    e. Attention to skin preparation and operative technique in addition to broad spectrum antibiotic prophylaxis are required to prevent graft infection

    f. Once infected a synthetic graft must usually be removed

    g. Recent reports have suggested that some infected grafts may be salvaged using antibiotic impregnated implants to provide a high local concentration of an appropriate antibiotic

3. Aneurysm

    a. Suture line aneurysms occur as a late complication

    b. Use of non-absorbable synthetic sutures such as prolene reduces the incidence of this complication

4. Graft failure

    a. Most early graft failures are related to technical errors

    b. Thrombosis is a common cause of early graft failure; graft thrombectomy or intra-arterial streptokinase may restore patency

    c. Progressive pseudointimal fibrous hyperplasia occurring at the site of arterial-graft anastomoses is an important cause of late graft occlusion especially if prosthetic materials are used

    d. Long-term graft patency can be improved by administering low-dose acetylsalicylic acid (aspirin) either alone or in combination with dipyridamole (Persantin)

Healing of synthetic arterial grafts

1. Endothelialisation from the adjacent host artery across the anastomotic line occurs to a maximum distance of 10 mm

2. Haematoma around the graft is organised by fibroblasts to form a surrounding capsule

3. Fibroblasts also grow through the interstices of the graft material to reach its luminal surface; grafts of high porosity allow greater ingrowth of fibroblasts

4. The luminal surface of the graft eventually consists of collagen fibres which are incompletely covered by endothelial cells

5. Seeding synthetic grafts with endothelial or mesothelial cells aims to reduce the thrombogenic potential of their luminal surface

FURTHER READING

Brewster D C, LaSalle A J, Robison J G, Strayhorn E C, Darling R C 1983, Factors affecting patency of femoropopliteal bypass grafts. Surg Gynecol Obstet 157: 437–442

Dardik H, Baier R E, Meenaghan M et al 1982 Morphologic and biophysical assessment of long term human umbilical cord vein implants used as vascular conduits. Surg Gynecol Obstet 154: 17–26

Goldman M D, Simpson D, Hawker R J, Norcott H C, McCollum C N 1983, Aspirin and dipyridamole reduce platelet deposition on prosthetic femoro-popliteal grafts in man. Ann Surg 198: 713–716

Green R M, Roedersheimer L R, DeWeese J A 1982 Effects of aspirin and dipyridamole on expanded polytetrafluoroethylene graft patency. Surgery 92: 1016–1026

Kidson I G 1983 Arterial prostheses. Br J Hosp Med 30: 248–254

McCollum C N 1986 In situ saphenous vein bypass. In Nyhus L N (ed) Surgery Annual Vol 18. Appleton-Century-Crofts, Norwalk, Connecticut pp 145–164 1986

McCollum C N 1985 Arterial bypass grafts for peripheral vascular disease. In: Taylor I (ed) Progress in Surgery Vol 1. Churchill Livingstone, Edinburgh pp 163–181

Raithel D, Schweinger H 1984 The Dardik biograft in reconstructive arterial surgery: report on a five year experience in 94 cases. World J Surg 8: 113–117

Smith S R G 1987 The principles underlying graft selection for arterial reconstruction. Br J Hosp Med 38: 358–363

Sterpetti A V, Schultz R D, Feldhaus R J, Peetz D J 1985 Seven-year experience with polytetrafluoroethylene as above-knee femoropoplital bypass graft. J Vasc Surg 2: 907–912

Umpleby H C, Britton D C, Turnbull A R 1987 Secondary arterio-enteric fistulae: a surgical challenge. Br J Surg 74: 256–259

ARTERIAL INJURY

Aetiology
1. Fractures
   a. Supracondylar fracture of humerus – brachial artery
   b. Fracture of clavicle or first rib – subclavian artery
   c. Fracture of shaft of femur – superficial femoral artery
2. Dislocation
   a. posterior dislocation of knee–popliteal artery
3. Penetrating injury
   a. Knife wound
   b. Missile injury; low velocity or high velocity
   c. Iatrogenic injury, e.g. operative wound, arterial cannulation for blood sampling, angiography or angioplasty
4. Blunt trauma
5. Crushing injury
6. Traction injury
   a. Over distraction of fractures during manipulation
   b. Injury to subclavian artery following acute lateral flexion of cervical spine
7. Acute deceleration injury
   a. Aortic tear at junction of aortic arch and descending thoracic aorta

8. Chemical injury
    a. Accidental intra-arterial injection of anaesthetic or sclerosant agents

Nature of arterial damage
1. Contusion of arterial wall
2. Stretching and spasm of arterial wall
3. Intimal tear with local or propagated thrombosis
4. Intimal flap with dissection and local or propagated thrombosis
5. Incomplete laceration of arterial wall which may be complicated by development of a false aneurysm. If there is simultaneous injury to an adjacent vein an arterio-venous fistula may form
6. Complete division of arterial wall
7. Loss of tissue of the arterial wall

Principles of management
1. Control haemorrhage and resuscitate patient
    a. Direct pressure is applied to the bleeding point
    b. Elevation of injured limb reduces both arterial and venous haemorrhage
    c. Tourniquets should only be used if absolutely necessary and must be applied correctly
    d. Intra-venous infusion of plasma expanders and blood is required in cases of significant blood loss
2. Signs of arterial occlusion indicate the need for urgent exploration
    a. Delay in revascularisation is associated with an increased rate of amputation
    b. Peripheral pulses may be palpable soon after trauma and their presence does not exclude arterial injury
    c. Delayed arterial occlusion may occur usually due to thrombosis
    d. Regular reassessment of the distal circulation is required for at least 24 hours following any possible arterial injury
3. In the absence of obvious clinical signs the diagnosis of arterial injury depends on a high index of suspicion
    a. The most subtle signs of distal ischaemia must be sought in the context of the nature and site of the proximal injury
    b. A distal pulse does not exclude the possibilty of arterial injury
    c. Arteriography should be performed early if suspicion exists
4. Penetrating injuries in the vicinity of major vessels should be explored even in the absence of signs of distal ischaemia to prevent formation of a false aneurysm or arterio-venous fistula
5. Arterial spasm should not be diagnosed unless structural arterial damage has been excluded by surgical exploration or a normal arteriogram

   a. Narrowing and loss of pulsation of an artery at the site of trauma is probably caused by intimal damage and thrombosis at that point rather than arterial spasm
   b. An arteriotomy at that point is required to determine the exact nature of the injury

Surgical principles
1. Prophylactic antibiotics are given if a penetrating wound is present or if prosthetic material is to be used
2. Tetanus prophylaxis is given if indicated
3. Before exposure of the damaged artery, control is obtained proximal and distal to the injured segment
4. Systemic heparin is given and the arterial tree distal to the injured segment is irrigated with heparinised saline
5. Proximal and distal catheter thrombectomy may be required to obtain good inflow and back-bleeding
6. Per-operative angiography may be required to determine the extent of the arterial injury or the presence of pre-existing occlusive arterial disease
7. Arterial repair
   a. Small clean lacerations of the arterial wall can often be closed primarily; a vein patch may be required to prevent excessive narrowing of the arterial lumen
   b. A severely contused or lacerated segment of artery should be excised: all damaged tissue should be removed
   c. Proximal and distal mobilisation of the artery may be sufficient to allow end-to-end anastomosis without tension but large collateral branches should not be divided
   d. If the cut ends of a damaged vessel cannot be apposed by direct suture without tension continuity is re-established by a reversed autogenous vein graft
   e. Prosthetic material such as Dacron may be required for the repair of larger arteries but should not be used in penetrating arterial injuries because of the danger of local sepsis and secondary haemorrhage
   f. Narrowing and loss of pulsation of an artery should not be considered to be due to spasm unless the vessel has been properly explored; arteriotomy should be performed and any intimal flaps sutured with fine sutures
   g. Genuine arterial spasm is treated by local application of papaverine
   h. If an arterio-venous fistula has formed the artery and vein are repaired and a muscle or fascial flap interposed between the two to prevent recurrence
8. Fasciotomy
   a. An essential adjunctive procedure in many cases of arterial injury especially those involving late re-vascularisation where gross swelling is likely to occur

    b. Subcutaneous fasciotomy via multiple small incisions often provides inadequate compartmental decompression

    c. For an adequate fasciotomy all fascial layers should be incised via a single longitudinal incision which is closed by delayed primary suture or skin grafting after 7–10 days when all oedema has subsided

9. Repair of venous injuries

    a. Every attempt should be made to repair injuries to major veins rather than employing simple ligation

    b. Venous thrombectomy may be required

10. Fracture stabilisation

    a. Simultaneous internal skeletal fixation is the ideal method of treating associated unstable fractures

    b. When wound contamination precludes its use skeletal traction or external skeletal fixation provide alternative methods

FURTHER READING

Kester R C, Leveson S H 1981 A Practice of Vascular Surgery. Pitman, London, pp 84–95

Meek A C, Robbs J V 1984 Vascular injury with associated bone and joint trauma. Br J Surg 71: 341–344

Sewell I A 1985 Recognition of arterial injury. Hosp Update 11: 209–216

Sewell I A 1985 Management of arterial injury. Hosp Update 11: 257–267

TRANSLUMINAL ANGIOPLASTY

Introduction

1. Transluminal angioplasty is a recently developed technique which is used to dilate arterial stenoses and recanalise short segments of occluded arteries

2. It may be used as an adjunct or alternative to conventional reconstructive vascular surgery, e.g. external iliac angioplasty prior to femoro-popliteal bypass grafting

3. Most commonly used to treat atheromatous disease but can also be used in cases of fibro-muscular dysplasia and neo-intimal hyperplasia

4. An increase in cross-sectional area of the treated artery is achieved by creating a longitudinal split through atheromatous plaques which separate from the media by local dissection and haemorrhage

5. Platelet and fibrin deposition followed by fibrosis later remodels the irregular area

Technique
1. The flexible double lumen polyvinyl catheter with a radio-opaque balloon (Gruntzig catheter) is inserted into the arterial lumen either percutaneously or at operation
2. Percutaneous transluminal angioplasty can be performed using local anaesthetic under light sedation
3. Following percutaneous puncture of a suitable artery (usually the common femoral) using the Seldinger technique, the balloon catheter is inserted over a guide wire under radiological control and positioned across the obstructing lesion
4. Heparin is injected intra-arterially and the balloon is then inflated to a predetermined pressure for 20–30 seconds
5. Effects of angioplasty can be assessed clinically and by comparison of pre- and post-dilatation angiograms or the pressure gradient across the lesion before and after its dilatation
6. Aspirin 75 mg twice daily or dipyridamole (Persantin) 100 mg three times daily is taken for at least 3 months following successful angioplasty to prevent reocclusion
7. All cases must be carefully selected and close cooperation between the vascular surgeon and the interventional radiologist is required for good results and the management of any complications which may develop

Indications
1. Peripheral vascular disease
   a. Isolated stenoses of the common and external iliac arteries
   b. Stenoses and short occlusions (<10 cm) of the superfical femoral and popliteal arteries
2. Renal artery stenosis
3. Coronary artery disease
   a. Localised strictures of the proximal part of a main coronary artery may be suitable for percutaneous angioplasty
   b. Other lesions especially those situated more distally may be suitable for dilatation at the time of coronary artery bypass grafting. See Page 149

Contra-indications
1. General
   a. Occluded vessel blocked flush with its origin
   b. No arterial lumen visualised distal to the obstruction
2. Specific
   a. Complete occlusion of aorta or iliac arteries
   b. Long occlusion (>10 cm) of superficial femoral artery

Complications
1. At the site of arterial puncture:
   a. Haemorrhage
   b. Haematoma
   c. False aneurysm

These complications can be reduced by application of adequate pressure after removal of the balloon catheter at the end of the procedure.

2. At the site of angioplasty:
   a. Subintimal arterial dissection
   b. Arterial perforation by guide-wire
   c. Arterial rupture
   d. Aneurysm formation
   e. Late reocclusion occurs in 40–60% of patients within 6 months depending on the site and nature of the lesion: antiplatelet agents can improve long-term patency results
3. Within the distal vasculature:
   a. Embolisation occurs in 5% of cases but is rarely of clinical significance.
   b. Arterial spasm
   c. Thrombosis

Advantages
1. Hospital stay of only 2–3 days and the low overall morbidity and mortality of percutaneous transluminal angioplasty compare favourably with those of conventional vascular surgical procedures
2. Can be used in elderly patients who present an unacceptably high risk for vascular reconstruction
3. Can be easily repeated at future dates if required
4. Reconstructive arterial surgery can be performed at a later date if necessary

FURTHER READING

Lamerton A 1986, Percutaneous transluminal angioplasty. Br J Surg 73: 91–97
Mosley J G, Raphael M 1986 Transluminal angioplasty. Hosp Update 12: 15–29
Petch M C 1987 Coronary angioplasty: a time for reappraisal. Br Med J 295: 453–454

ABDOMINAL AORTIC ANEURYSMS

Abdominal aortic aneurysms are four times more common in men than women and their incidence appears to be increasing in both sexes. They account for just over 1% of all deaths in men over 65 years in this country.

Indications for surgery
1. Emergency surgery
   a. Extraperitoneal rupture produces an expanding retroperitoneal haematoma contained by the posterior parietal peritoneum
   b. Intraperitoneal rupture leads to rapid and massive blood loss which is usually immediately fatal
2. Early surgery
   a. Abdominal or lumbar pain indicate rapid expansion of the aneurysm which is tender on clinical examination; these features indicate imminent rupture
   b. Peripheral embolisation
3. Elective surgery
   a. Asymptomatic aneursyms are discovered by abdominal palpation, plain abdominal radiography, ultrasonography or computed tomography
   b. Elective repair is usually offered to patients under 75 years with asymptomatic aneurysms greater than 5 cm in diameter provided they are fit for major surgery

Surgical repair
1. Antibiotic prophylaxis to prevent septic complications is started pre-operatively and continued for 48–72 hours
2. Full-length midline abdominal incision: most aortic aneurysms arise below the renal arteries and are accessible via this incision
3. Peritoneum over the aneurysmal sac is incised and the duodenum mobilised: along with the small intestine it is displaced to the right
4. Aneurysms may be adherent to the inferior vena cava, left renal vein, or common iliac veins which may all be damaged during the dissection to obtain proximal and distal control. Adherence to the duodeno-jejunal flexure may also occur
5. Left renal vein may be divided between ligatures to improve access to the aorta proximal to the aneurysm
6. Dacron graft is pre-clotted prior to heparinisation of the patient
7. After cross-clamping the aorta and common iliac arteries the aneurysm sac is opened longitudinally. Blood, blood clot and atheromatous material are evacuated. Excision of the sac is unnecessary and liable to damage adjacent structures and increase operative blood loss
8. Lumbar arteries are oversewn with non-absorbable sutures
9. If the common iliac arteries are not dilated the aneurysm can be repaired using a straight tube graft inlayed into the sac. By reducing the number of vascular anastomoses operating time is minimised. Significant dilatation of the iliac arteries requires the use of an aorto-iliac or aorto-femoral bifurcation graft, the proximal ends of the iliac arteries having been ligated or oversewn

10. Bifurcation grafts should be sutured under light tension and have a short stem to ensure an acute angle between the bifurcating limbs which will prevent kinking at the bifurcation
11. Backflow from the distal arteries should be checked before completing the distal anastomoses and Fogarty embolectomy catheters passed if necessary
12. Slow and intermittent release of cross-clamps prevents sudden and profound hypotension due to anoxic vasodilatation in the lower limbs and metabolic acidosis which is caused by the rapid release of products of anaerobic metabolism into the systemic circulation
13. The remainder of the aneurysm sac is wrapped over the graft especially at the suture lines to prevent adherence to the adjacent duodenum and small intestine and possible aorto-enteric fistulation

Complications of aortic aneurysm repair
1. Haemorrhage
2. Shock
3. Renal failure
4. Cardiac failure
5. Peripheral embolisation
6. Graft occlusion
7. Colonic ischaemia
8. Aorto-enteric fistula
9. Anastomotic aneurysm

Mortality of aortic aneurysm repair
1. Elective surgery should be associated with a mortality below 5%
2. The mortality of emergency surgery remains about 40–60%
3. Operative mortality of emergency repair is increased by the following factors:
   a. Advanced age
   b. Pre-operative hypotension
   c. Extensive pre-operative haemorrhage
   d. Large volumes of pre- and post-operative blood transfusion
4. The exact mortality figures of each surgical department are also influenced by patient selection
5. Patients who survive repair of an aortic aneurysm should have a normal life expectancy

FURTHER READING

Campbell W B, Collin J, Morris P J 1986 The mortality of abdominal aortic aneurysm. Ann R Coll Surg Eng 68: 275–278
Castleden W M, Mercer J C 1985 Abdominal aortic aneurysms in Western

Australia: descriptive epidemiology and patterns of rupture. Br J Surg
72: 109–112

Collin J 1985 Screening for abdominal aortic aneurysms. Br J Surg
72: 851–852

Gardham J R C 1982 Abdominal aortic aneurysms. Br J Hosp Med
28: 40–47

Makin G S 1983 Changing fashions in the surgery of aortic aneurysms. Ann
R Coll Surg Eng 65: 308–310

Sewell I A 1985 Arterial emergencies: aneurysms. Hosp Update 11: 517–532

SURGERY FOR CEREBRAL ISCHAEMIA

Introduction

1. In many patients with cerebro-vascular insufficiency the atherosclerotic stenosis or occlusion involves the extra-cranial arteries, is segmental rather than diffuse and may be amenable to surgical correction
2. The majority of surgically correctable lesions are at the bifurcation of the common carotid artery. All three carotid arteries are usually involved but the common carotid artery often occludes first and blood flow through the internal carotid artery may be maintained by retrograde filling from the external carotid artery
3. Correctable lesions of the brachio-cephalic, subclavian, and vertebral arteries are less commonly found. As there is usually abundant collateral flow following occlusion of one of the major arterial trunks, multiple lesions are normally present by the time symptoms appear
4. When extra-cranial surgery is not possible, usually because of occlusion of the internal carotid artery, the patient may be suitable for intra-cranial revascularisation from one of the extra-cranial arteries

Clinical features

Symptoms of cerebro-vascular insufficiency are due either to embolisation of platelet aggregates or atheromatous debris from ulcerated atherosclerotic plaques or to reduction in cerebral blood flow as a result of occlusive arterial disease.

1. Hypoperfusion of the carotid artery territory
   a. Ipsilateral visual disturbance including blurring of vision and temporary visual field loss (amaurosis fugax)
   b. Contralateral motor or sensory impairment
   c. Dysphasia if dominant hemisphere affected
2. Hypoperfusion of vertebro-basilar artery territory
   a. Visual disturbances including diplopia and homonymous hemianopia
   b. Ataxia
   c. Syncopal (drop) attacks

Indications for surgical treatment
1. Transient ischaemic attacks (TIAs)
   a. A TIA is characterised by focal neurological symptoms and signs of less than 24 hours duration and not associated with any subsequent neurological deficit
   b. Strokes occur in 7% of patients within one year of their first TIA
   c. Surgical treatment is designed to prevent irreversible cerebro-vascular accidents
   d. Symptomatic patients with greater than 50–70% carotid stenosis are usually considered for surgical treatment
2. Asymtomatic carotid bruits are rarely an indication for surgery as the risk of stroke in these patients is only 1% per year
3. Rarely a slowly evolving ('stuttering') stroke may be an indication for surgery

Contra-indications to surgical treatment
1. Dense acute completed stroke
2. Rapidly progressing or rapidly improving strokes
3. Advanced biological age
4. Severe coronary arterial disease
5. Marked hypertension
6. Generalised intra-cranial and extra-cranial arterial disease

Investigations and pre-operative assessment
In addition to the usual routine investigations performed on all patients with degenerative arterial disease patients with cerebro-vascular disease undergo the following pre-operative tests. Non-invasive investigations are performed prior to invasive angiography which is reserved for those patients likely to undergo surgery. Despite improved techniques invasive arteriography is still associated with a small risk of stroke.
1. Continuous wave Doppler imaging with spectrum analysis
2. Pulsed Doppler imaging – Mobile artery and vein imaging system (MAVIS)
3. Real-time B-mode ultra-sonographic scanning
4. Duplex ultrasound (B-mode ultrasonography combined with pulsed Doppler imaging)
5. Intra-venous digital subtraction arteriography (DSA)
6. Conventional arteriography
   a. Trans-femoral arch aortography and selective vessel arteriography
   b. Direct carotid arteriography

Other investigations which have been used in the assessment of patients with cerebral ischaemia include oculo-plethysmography (OPG), spectral analysis carotid phono-angiography (CPA) and supra-orbital Doppler examination.

Surgical treatment

1. Carotid bifurcation endarterectomy
   a. Indicated in the presence of an ulcerating non-stenosing atheromatous plaque or stenosis of the internal carotid artery reducing its luminal diameter to less than 50%
   b. Usually performed under general anaesthesia although local anaesthetic techniques may be used
   c. A longitudinal arteriotomy in the common carotid artery is extended into the internal carotid artery
   d. A silastic intra-luminal (Javid) shunt may be inserted into the common carotid artery proximally and the internal carotid artery distally to preserve the cerebral blood flow. Some surgeons use it routinely, others only on a selective basis if the stump systolic pressure is less than 50 mm Hg or in the presence of vertebral arterial or contra-lateral carotid arterial disease or if pre-operative EEG changes occur
   e. Hypothermia can provide further protection against the effects of per-operative cerebral ischaemia
   f. The carotid sinus nerve is often blocked using local anaesthetic but is not usually divided
   g. After endartectomy is completed the distal intima may need to be fixed with fine axial sutures to prevent dissection
   h. Closure of the arteriotomy is usually performed using sutures and rarely requires the use of a vein patch
   i. The operative mortality should be less than 2%; approximately 1–2% of patients will develop a stroke following carotid endarterectomy
   j. About 1% of patients suffering TIAs and undergoing carotid endarterectomy can be expected to develop a significant stroke in each of the following years; in contrast 5–7% of similar patients not treated surgically will develop a stroke each year
2. Surgical treatment of lesions of other extra-cranial arteries
   a. Single occlusions of the proximal part of the subclavian artery causing subclavian steal syndrome can be bypassed using axillo-axillary, subclavian-subclavian or carotid-subclavian grafts provided the other major vessels are relatively free of disease. In this way the need for intra-thoracic surgery is avoided
   b. Multiple stenotic lesions of the origins of the innominate, left common carotid and left subclavian arteries require extensive reconstruction of the aortic arch and its major branches
   c. Vertebral endarterectomy can be performed via a medial supra-clavicular approach; access to the origin of the vertebral artery is through a short subclavian arteriotomy

3. Extra-cranial intra-cranial revascularisation
   a. Indicated when distal internal carotid artery occlusion
      precludes carotid bifurcation endarterectomy and other
      forms of vascular reconstruction are not feasible
   b. A suitable scalp artery, usually the anterior branch of the
      superfical temporal artery, is mobilised from the deep
      surface of a widely based lateral scalp flap
   c. A 5 cm diameter craniectomy is fashioned and the dura
      incised
   d. Microvascular techniques are used to anastomose the
      mobilised scalp vessel end-to-side to an appropriate cortical
      branch of the middle cerebral artery
   e. In patients with symptoms of vertebro-basilar insufficiency
      the occipital artery can be anastomosed to the posterior
      inferior cerebellar artery through a small occipital
      craniectomy
   f. It is claimed that the increased cerebral blood flow is
      associated with reduction in the incidence of TIAs and
      strokes

FURTHER READING

Caplan L R 1986 Carotid artery disease. New Eng J Med 315: 886–868
Chambers B R, Norris J W 1986 Outcome in patients with asymptomatic
    neck bruits. N Eng J Med 315: 860–865
Colgan M P, Kingston W, Shanik D G 1985 Asymptomatic carotid stenosis:
    is prophylactic endarterectomy justifiable? Br J Surg 72: 313–314
Eastcott H H G 1986 Carotid endarterectomy: a mid-atlantic view. Br J Surg
    73: 865–866
Ellis M, Dain R M, Greenhalgh R M 1987 The clinical value of noninvasive
    assessment of the carotid arteries. Hosp Update 13: 627–638
Kester R C, Leveson S H 1981 A Practice of Vascular Surgery Pitman,
    London pp 151–190
Lawson L J 1981 Surgery for extracranial carotid artery disease. Hosp
    Update 7: 899–904
Murie J A, Morris P J 1986 Carotid endarterectomy in Great Britain and
    Ireland. Br J Surg 73: 867–870
Myers K A, Nicolaides A N 1986 New developments in arterial surgery.
    Recent Advances in Surgery Vol 12. In: Russell R C G (ed) Churchill
    Livingstone, Edinburgh pp 251–269
Thompson J E 1983 Carotid endarterectomy, 1982 – the state of the art. Br J
    Surg 70: 371–376

SURGERY FOR MYOCARDIAL ISCHAEMIA

Coronary artery surgery has been performed on an increasing
number of patients over the last 15 years. Its indications have
increased and it is now one of the commonest surgical operations
performed in the USA.

Techniques
1. Reversed autogenous vein aorto-coronary artery bypass graft
   a. For individual vein grafts separate lengths of saphenous vein are anastomosed end-to-side to the ascending aorta and end-to-side to each coronary artery distal to the obstructing lesion
   b. With 'jump grafts' a single saphenous vein graft is used to feed several coronary arteries via a series of side-to-side anastomoses
   c. If the long saphenous vein is not available due to previous excision or injection of sclerosants the cephalic vein can be used but it is a poor substitute
2. Coronary artery endarterectomy
   a. This often performed in conjunction with bypass grafting at the site of the arteriotomy
   b. Used on its own this procedure gives poor results
3. Internal mammary (thoracic) artery transfer
   a. The internal mammary artery is mobilised from the anterior chest wall
   b. It is used either as a free graft or a sequential graft to the coronary artery
4. Transluminal angioplasty
   a. Small vessels may be dilated using a balloon catheter introduced via an arteriotomy at the time of bypass surgery
   b. Percutaneous transluminal angioplasty is being increasingly used especially in the treatment of recurrent symptoms after coronary artery bypass grafting

Indications
1. Relief of ischaemic symptoms
   a. Stable angina which is disabling and refractory to full medical treatment irrespective of the number and site of coronary arterial stenoses
   b. Unstable angina unresponsive to conventional medical treatment in patients with critical stenoses of one or more coronary arteries
2. Improve the prognosis of young patients with ischaemic heart disease
   a. Triple vessel disease
   b. Left main stem stenosis
3. Acute myocardial infarction
   a. Caused by dissection of a coronary artery at coronary arteriography
   b. As a complication of percutaneous transluminal balloon catheter angioplasty
   c. Refractory cardiogenic shock requiring use of an intra-aortic balloon counter-pulsation pump
   d. Selected cases of spontaneous acute myocardial infarction with significant multiple vessel disease

4. In association with aortic valve replacement
   a. If severe coronary artery stenoses are present coronary artery bypass grafting should be considered at the time of aortic valve replacement
   b. It does not increase operative mortality and grafting may improve the long-term prognosis in these patients
5. In association with other surgical procedures for the treatment of complications of ischaemic heart disease
   a. Mitral valve replacement following papillary muscle rupture
   b. Repair of acquired ventricular septal defect
   c. Resection of left ventricular aneurysm

Contra-indications
1. Advanced age
2. Other diseases limiting life expectancy
3. Widespread coronary arterial disease
4. Poor run-off distal to occluded or stenosed segments
5. Excessive myocardial damage with poor left ventricular function (ejection fraction less than 20 per cent)

Results
1. Operative morbidity
   a. Peri-operative infarction occurs in 5% of cases as indicated by ECG changes and elevation of cardiac enzymes; although rarely fatal it is associated with an increased rate of complications and impaired long-term prognosis
   b. Cerebral complications are thought to be secondary to cardio-pulmonary bypass or emboli of atheromatous material
   c. Disruption of the median sternotomy wound occurs in 1–2% of cases
   d. Infection or distruption of the leg wound through which the saphenous vein is harvested occurs rarely
2. Operative mortality
   a. For patients with uncomplicated chronic myocardial ischaemia the operative mortality rate should be less than 2.5%
   b. Operative mortality is increased in those over 65 years.
   c. Women have a risk more than twice that of men
   d. Other factors associated with increased mortality include:
      (i) impaired left ventricular function
      (ii) recent myocardial infarction
      (iii) excision of left ventricular aneurysm
      (iv) repair of septal defects
3. Relief of symptoms
   a. Up to 90% of patients with angina should experience complete relief of pain which is maintained for at least one year in most cases; 50% remain asymptomatic after 10 years

b. 60–90% of patients will be able to resume full-time employment
4. Graft patency
   a. 80% of vein grafts are patent at 3 years
   b. 10% of grafts occlude in the first two post-operative weeks
   c. Long-term patency can be improved by routine use of dipyridamole or aspirin
5. Long-term survival
   a. Results from prospective randomised trials show that patients with left main stem coronary artery disease have a 93% 5-year survival rate if treated surgically compared to only 62% in those treated medically
   b. Patients with triple vessel disease having bypass surgery have a 5-year survival rate of 95% compared with 85% in patients having conventional medical treatment
   c. Improved survival in patients undergoing coronary artery bypass surgery is still evident after 10 years

FURTHER READING

Brooks N 1983 Indications for coronary artery surgery. J R Coll Phys 22: 23–27
Ross J K 1985 Surgery for myocardial ischaemia. In: Taylor I (ed) Progress in Surgery Vol 1., Churchill Livingstone, Edinburgh pp 147–162
Raphael M J, Donaldson R M 1985 Coronary transluminal angioplasty. Br J Hosp Med 33: 18–22
Reeder G S, Krishan I, Nobrega F T et al 1984 Is percutaneous coronary angioplasty less expensive than bypass surgery. New Eng J Med 311: 1157–1162
Treasure T 1983 Coronary artery bypass surgery. Br J Hosp Med 30: 259–263
Treasure T 1987 Hearts and minds; how big is the risk of coronary artery surgery. Br J Hosp Med 37: 9

POST-OPERATIVE DEEP VEIN THROMBOSIS AND PULMONARY EMBOLISM

If no prophylactic measures are taken deep vein thrombosis (DVT) will be seen in up to 50% of patients undergoing major abdominal, pelvic or hip surgery. 20% of those patients with a deep vein thrombosis are at risk of developing a pulmonary embolism (PE).

Pathogenesis of deep vein thrombosis (Virchow's triad)
1. Alteration of venous blood flow
   a. Stasis
   b. Turbulence
2. Endothelial damage

  3. Alteration of blood constituents
     a. Increased platelet adhesiveness
     b. Activation of procoagulants
An aggregate of platelets with fibrin deposition produces a stable nidus of thrombus. If this is not cleared the thrombus is readily propagated.

Predisposing factors
  1. Previous deep vein thrombosis or pulmonary embolism
  2. Varicose veins
  3. Oestrogen therapy and oral contraceptives
  4. Pregnancy and puerperium
  5. Obesity
  6. Elderly patients
  7. Malignant disease
  8. Prolonged immobilisation
  9. Extensive burns and trauma, especially pelvic and femoral fractures
 10. Major surgery, especially abdominal and pelvic operations
 11. Blood group A
 12. Increased euglobulin lysis time (ELT)
 13. Reduced anti-thrombin III concentration
 14. Myocardial infarction
 15. Congestive cardiac failure

Diagnosis of deep vein thrombosis
  1. History and clinical examination
     a. Both are very unreliable
     b. Classical presentation is quite rare
     c. Many patients with established venous thromboses are asymptomatic
     d. Most patients have non-specific or equivocal physical signs
  2. Radio-active (^{125}I-labelled) fibrinogen uptake
     a. Only detects developing thrombi
     b. Very sensitive method below the knee with an accuracy of 80–90%
     c. Unreliable in the upper thigh
     d. Cannot be used for pelvic vein thromboses
     e. False positive results occur in the presence of haematomata or recent surgical or traumatic wounds
     f. Useful tool for research investigations and as a routine screening test in high-risk patients
  3. Contrast venography
     a. Provides the 'gold standard' against which other tests are compared
     b. Usually performed to confirm the diagnosis of deep vein thrombosis
     c. Accurately documents the extent of a thrombus and its nature

   d. Ascending venography is used to show the calf and thigh veins; per-trochanteric injection may be used to demonstrate thrombi in the pelvic veins

   e. An expensive and time consuming investigation

   f. May be complicated by allergic reactions, thrombophlebitis and thrombosis

4. Radio-nuclide venography
   a. Very expensive technique requiring specialised equipment and skilled staff
   b. Suitable for detecting thrombi above the knee
   c. Relatively free of complications

5. Doppler ultrasonography
   a. Practical technique using easily portable and relatively inexpensive equipment
   b. Absence of ionising radiation allows its use in pregnancy
   c. May not detect non-occlusive thrombi which do not significantly alter the dynamics of venous flow
   d. Presence of occlusive thrombi may be masked by flow in collateral or superficial veins
   e. Overall accuracy is 85%, being greater for ilio-femoral than tibio-popliteal thromboses
   f. Widely used as a screening technique

6. Thermography
   a. Infra-red camera detects areas of increased temperature
   b. In the absence of inflammatory conditions these areas are related to the presence of an underlying thrombus

7. Strain guage and impedance plethysmography
   a. Plethysmographic techniques measure the venous volume of the lower limb and venous emptying time
   b. Suitable for detecting major proximal venous occlusion

Prophylaxis against deep vein thrombosis

All patients at high risk should receive some form of prophylaxis and be routinely screened for the presence of asymptomatic deep vein thromboses.

Mechanical methods
1. Static graduated compression of legs
   a. Thrombo-embolic deterrent (TED) stockings
   b. Decopress thrombosis prophylactic stockings
   c. Thrombex anti-embolism stockings

2. Electrical calf muscle stimulation
   a. Powley–Doran electronic gaiters
   b. Thrombophylactor gaiters

3. Passive exercise of legs
   a. Physiotherapy
   b. Foot pedalling machine

4. Intermittent external pneumatic compression of legs
    a. Flowtron boots
    b. Roberts venous flow stimulator
    c. Kendall sequential compression device

Chemical methods
1. Heparin
    a. Low dose subcutaneous calcium or sodium heparin (5000 units 8- or 12-hourly) is given pre-operatively and continued for 5–7 days
    b. Low molecular weight heparin has less risk of haemorrhage than unfractionated heparin
    c. Ultra-low dose intra-venous heparin (1 unit/kg body weight per hour) administered by infusion pump for 3–5 days
2. Dihydroergotamine
    a. An ergot alkaloid which acts as an α-adrenergic receptor stimulant to increase the muscular tone of the vein walls
    b. Administered subcutaneously (0.5 mg 8-hourly) and usually used in conjuction with low dose heparin
3. Platelet inhibitory agents, e.g. aspirin, dipyridamole, sulphinpyrazone, Dextran 70
    a. Have fewer haemorrhagic problems than anticoagulants
    b. Occasional anaphylactoid reactions to Dextran can be avoided by prior infusion of a hapten
4. Oral anticoagulant, e.g. warfarin, phenindione
    a. These drugs need strict laboratory control and are incompatible with a number of other drugs
    b. Significant haemorrhage may occur and the effects of these anticoagulants may be difficult to reverse

No method of prophylaxis either chemical or mechanical is 100% effective: in very high risk patients a mechanical method should therefore be combined with a chemical one.

Treatment of established deep vein thrombosis
1. Bed rest
2. Leg elevation
3. Compression of affected leg
    a. Conventional bandaging
    b. Graded compression stockings
4. Anticoagulants
    a. Full anticoagulation is achieved with heparin given by continuous intra-venous infusion for at least 5 days
    b. Warfarin is then given for 3–6 months in most cases
5. Fibrinolysis
    a. Urokinase is a very expensive plasminogen activator derived from human urine
    b. Streptokinase is much cheaper but is associated with allergic reactions; anaphylaxis may occur

6. Vein ligation and venous thrombectomy
   a. Indicated in the presence of severe ilio-femoral venous thrombosis with impending venous gangrene which does not respond to anticoagulants and where fibrinolytic agents are contraindicated
   b. Ilio-femoral venous thrombectomy may be combined with ligation of the superficial femoral vein

Diagnosis of pulmonary embolism
1. History and clinical examination
   a. Only one third of patients with clinical features compatible with a major pulmonary embolus have the diagnosis confirmed by angiography
   b. Similarly pulmonary embolus is often not diagnosed as it is clinically silent or its presentation atypical
2. Chest radiography
   A number of abnormalities may be present but none is specific for pulmonary embolus
   a. Areas of decreased and increased pulmonary vascular markings
   b. Prominent hilar shadow
   c. Pulmonary atelectasis or consolidation
   d. Pleural effusion
   e. Elevated hemi-diaphragm
3. Electrocardiogram (ECG)
   a. Massive pulmonary embolus is associated with signs of acute right ventricular strain
   b. Typical ECG features include 'S1, Q3, T3' pattern with T wave inversion in leads V1–V3
4. Arterial blood gas analysis
   a. Low arterial oxygen tension
   b. Low arterial carbon dioxide tension
5. Radio-isotope ventilation-perfusion lung scintigraphy
   a. The regional distribution of inhaled radio-active gas (^{81}Kr) is compared with the distribution of radio-labelled particles (^{99}Tc-labelled macroaggregates of albumin) injected intra-venously
   b. Pulmonary emboli produce perfusion defects which are not associated with corresponding ventilation defects
6. Pulmonary angiography
   a. Definitive method of diagnosing pulmonary embolism
   b. The extent and site of the obstruction to the pulmonary circulation is determined and the age of the embolus can be estimated

Treatment of pulmonary embolism
1. Immediate resuscitation
   a. External cardiac massage
   b. Endotracheal intubation
   c. Oxygen
   d. 8.4% Sodium bicarbonate infusion to reverse metabolic acidosis
2. Anticoagulants
   a. Heparin is given intra-venously in the acute stage
   b. Warfarin is prescribed after a few days and the patient normally maintained on oral anticoagulants for at least 3–6 months
3. Plasminogen activators
   a. Streptokinase and urokinase can be used to accelerate the clearance of pulmonary emboli in the initial 24 hours
   b. The efficacy of these thrombolysins is increased by their direct infusion into the pulmonary arteries via the catheter used for initial arteriography
4. Pulmonary embolectomy
   a. Open embolectomy (Trendelenburg's operation) ideally using cardio-pulmonary bypass but if this is not available an attempt can be made using the normothermic venous inflow occlusion technique
   b. Catheter embolectomy using a steerable cup-catheter inserted via the femoral or internal jugular vein and guided under flouroscopic control

Prevention of pulmonary embolism in patients with established deep vein thrombosis
1. Anticoagulants
   a. Heparin
   b. Warfarin
2. Plasminogen activators
   a. Streptokinase
   b. Urokinase
3. Defibrinating agents
   a. Ancrod (Arvin) is an enzyme derived from the venom of the Malayan pit viper
   b. Given subcutaneously or intra-venously it lowers serum fibrinogen levels by cleaving fibrinopeptide A from fibrinogen
   c. Fibrinogen degradation products which are formed have significant anticoagulant activity
4. Venous thrombectomy
5. Inferior vena caval ligation or plication
6. Trans-venous insertion of intra-caval device
   a. Used for patients with recurrent pulmonary emboli in whom anticoagulants are either contra-indicated or ineffective

b. Can be inserted under local anaesthesia and is now used in preference to vena caval ligation or plication
c. Inserted via the internal jugular or femoral vein and usually placed just below the renal veins
d. Examples of the devices commonly used include the Mobin–Uddin umbrella filter, Kimray-Greenfield wire filter, Eichelter sieve and Pate clip

FURTHER READING

Colditz G A, Tuden R L, Oster G 1986 Rates of venous thrombosis after general surgery: combined results of randomised clinical trials. Lancet ii: 143–146

Comerota A J, White J V, Katz M L 1985 Diagnostic methods for deep vein thrombosis: Venous Doppler examination, phleborheography, iodine-125 fibrinogen uptake and phlebography. Am J Surg 150: 14–24

Consensus Conference 1986 Prevention of venous thrombosis and pulmonary embolism. J A M A 256: 744–749

Coon W W 1977 Epidemiology of venous thromboembolism. Ann Surg 186: 149–164

Dalen J E, Paraskos J A, Ockene I S, Alpert J S, Hirsh J 1986 Venous thromboembolism. Scope of the problem. Chest 89 (Suppl): S370–373

Greenfield L J, Langham M R 1984 Surgical approaches to thrombo-embolism. Br J Surg 71: 968–970

Hedges A R, Kakkar V V 1988 Prophylaxis of pulmonary embolism and deep vein thrombosis. Hosp Update 14: 1159–1174

Hull R D, Raskob G E, Hirsh J 1986 Prophylaxis of venous thromboembolism. An overview. Chest 89 (Suppl): S374–383

Ruckley C V 1985 Protection against thrombo-embolism. Br. J Surg 72: 421–422

Russell J C 1983 Prophylaxis of postoperative deep vein thrombosis and pulmonary embolism. Surg Gynecol Obstet 157: 89–104

Salzman E W, Davies G C 1980 Prophylaxis of venous thromboembolism. Analysis of cost effectiveness. Ann Surg 191: 207–208

Scurr J H, Jarrett P E M, Wastell C 1983 The treatment of recurrent pulmonary embolism: experience with the Kimray Greenfield vena cava filter. Ann R Coll Surg Eng 65: 233–234

Sue-Ling M H, Johnston D, McMahon M J, Philips P R, Davies J A 1986 Pre-operative identification of patients at high risk of deep venous thrombosis after major abdominal surgery. Lancet i: 1173–1176

Organ transplantation

TRANSPLANTATION AND IMMUNOSUPPRESSION

Transplantation antigens
1. Histocompatibility antigens are genetically determined and therefore specific to each individual
2. The histocompatibility antigens are present on the surface of nucleated cells within the body and are known as human leucocyte-associated antigens (HLA antigens)
3. These are controlled by the major histocompatibility (MHC) complex which is located on the short arms of chromosome 6
4. Class I HLA antigens are found on the surface of most cells within the body and controlled by the loci designated A, B and C
5. Class II HLA antigens are controlled by loci in the D region and have a more restricted expression than Class I antigens; they are found on dendritic cells, B lymphocytes and activated T cells
6. The HLA system is the most polymorphic genetic system in man, 8–40 different antigens having been identified at each locus
7. The potential number of different phenotypes is therefore extremely large and in practice only identical twins have identical patterns of HLA antigens
8. For practical purposes in organ transplantation serological typing can be performed for the A and B loci (Class I) and the DR locus (Class II)

Selection of donors
1. Most cadaver organs come from donors who have suffered irreversible structural brain damage following road traffic accidents or cerebro-vascular catastrophes and been diagnosed as 'Brain Dead'
2. Age: For renal donors <70 years; For other organs <30 years
3. Satisfactory renal, cardiac, pancreatic or hepatic function is required
4. No evidence of systemic infection especially hepatitis-B and HTLV-III (HIV) viruses

5. No evidence of malignant disease except for primary central nervous system tumours
6. ABO blood group compatibility is essential for all transplants
7. HLA antigen compatibility plays a significant role in donor selection for most forms of organ allograft
   a. The A, B and DR antigens of the potential donor are identified by incubating donor lymphocytes with a range of HLA typing sera
   b. Compatibility at the DR and B loci have the greatest influence on graft survival
8. Kidney transplants from live-related donors can also be considered as the results are generally better than those from cadaver donors. The results with organs from HLA identical siblings are particularly good

Non-specific immunosuppressive agents
1. Cortico-steroids
   Steroids, such as prednisolone exert powerful immunosuppressive as well as anti-inflammatory actions, and are widely used in maintenance immunosuppresive regimens and to treat acute rejection episodes. They have several useful actions:
   a. Decrease macrophage activity, motility and phagocytic activity
   b. Reduce circulating T-cell populations
   c. Depress T-cell response to mitogens
   d. Stabilise lysosomal and cellular membranes
   e. Inhibit release of vasoactive amines and proteolytic enzymes
2. Azathioprine and 6-mercaptopurine
   a. Azathioprine is metabolised to 6-mercatopurine within the liver
   b. 6-mercaptopurine acts as a purine antagonist reducing the synthesis of DNA and RNA by dividing cells
   c. This causes impairment of IgG production by B-cells and inhibition of killer T-cells
3. Cyclophosphamide
   a. Inert agent activated by hepatic microsomal enzymes to produce several alkylating metabolites
   b. Active metabolites cause cross-links between DNA strands preventing division of immunocompetent cells
4. Cyclosporin
   a. Cyclical polypeptide comprising 11 amino acids and originally produced by a cell fungus, Trichoderma polysporum
   b. Fat soluble, water insoluble
   c. Acts at an intra-cellular level to block the proliferation of cytotoxic T-lymphocytes

5. Anti-lymphocyte (ALG) and anti-thymocyte (ATG) globulins
   a. Derived from anti-serum to human lymphocytes and thymocytes prepared in foreign species
   b. Deplete circulating T-lymphocytes and lymphocytes within lymphoid organs

Other immunosuppressive techniques
1. Irradiation
   a. Whole body
   b. Total lymphoid
   c. Allograft
   d. Peripheral blood (extra-corporeal)
2. Thymectomy
3. Thoracic duct drainage
4. Splenectomy
5. Plasmapheresis

Complications of immunosuppressive agents
Until donor-specific immunosuppressive techniques can be safely applied in the clinical situation non-specific immunosuppressive agents will continue to be used. The most serious complication of non-specific immunosuppression is an increased susceptibility to various infections:
1. Bacterial, e.g.
   a. *Listeria monocytogenes*
   b. *Mycobacterium tuberculosis*
2. Fungal, e.g.
   a. *Candida albicans*
   b. Histoplasmosis
   c. Aspergillosis
   d. *Nocardia asteroides*
   e. *Cryptococcus neoformans*
3. Protozoal, e.g.
   a. *Pneumocystis carinii*
   b. Cryptosporidiosis
4. Viral, e.g.
   a. Cytomegalovirus (CMV)
   b. Epstein–Barr virus (EBV)
   c. Herpes simplex
   d. Herpes zoster
   e. Measles

Transplant recipients also have an increased susceptibility to various neoplasms:
1. Malignant lymphoma
2. Skin tumours
3. Malignancy transferred with the donor organ

Other complications are related to specific immunosuppressive agents:

1. Corticosteroids, e.g. prednisolone, methylprednisolone
   a. Impaired growth
   b. Wound infection and impaired wound healing
   c. Osteoporosis
   d. Avascular bone necrosis
   e. Acute pancreatitis
   f. Diabetes mellitus
   g. Cataracts
   h. Peptic ulceration
   i. Hypertension
   j. Psychosis
2. Antimetabolites, e.g. azathioprine, 6-mercaptopurine,
   a. Myelosuppresion
   b. Hepatotoxicity
   c. Cholestatic jaundice
   d. Acute pancreatitis
3. Alkylating agents, e.g. cyclophosphamide
   a. Myelosuppression
   b. Haemorrhagic cystitis
   c. Nausea and vomiting
   d. Alopecia
   e. Sterility
4. Anti-lymphocyte and anti-thymocyte globulins (ALG and ATG)
   a. Painful indurated injection sites
   b. Anaphylaxis
   c. Arthus phenomenom
5. Cyclosporin
   a. Nephrotoxicity
   b. Hepatotoxicity
   c. Gingival hypertrophy
   d. Hypertrichosis

FURTHER READING

Amlot P L 1982 The side effects of immunosuppression. Hosp Update
    8: 1007–1012
Cameron S 1982 Immunosuppression after transplantation. Hosp Update
    8: 835–848
Dick H M 1983 Role of HL-A system in graft rejection. Hosp Update
    9: 415–426
Van Buren C T 1986 Cyclosporine: progress, problems and perspectives.
    Surg Clin N Am 66: 435–450
Salaman J R 1983 Steroids and modern immunosuppression. Br Med J
    286: 1373–1375
Salaman J R 1982 Non-specific immunosuppression. In: Morris P J (ed)
    Clinical Surgery International Vol 3 Tissue Transplantation. Churchill
    Livingstone, Edinburgh pp 60–79
Ting A 1982 HLA and organ transplantation. In: Morris P J (ed) Clinical
    Surgery International Vol 3 Tissue Transplantation. Churchill Livingstone,
    Edinburgh pp 28–39

RENAL TRANSPLANTATION

Renal transplantation is the most acceptable form of treatment for end-stage renal failure. More than 12,000 renal transplants are now performed annually throughout the world.

Indications
Renal transplantation is indicated in the treatment of end-stage renal failure due to a wide range of conditions:
1. Chronic glomerulonephritis
2. Chronic pyelonephritis
3. Malignant hypertension
4. Polycystic disease
5. Diabetic nephropathy
6. Analgesic nephropathy

Contra-indications
1. Unacceptable operative risk due to severe coincident cardio-pulmonary disease
2. Disseminated malignant disease

Operative technique

Donor operation
1. Living-related donor nephrectomy is performed through a standard loin incision
2. En bloc removal of the kidneys in cadaver donor nephrectomy minimises the risk of damage to accessory renal vessels
3. Cadaver donor nephrectomy prior to cardio-respiratory arrest minimises the warm ischaemia time
4. Following its removal the kidney is perfused intra-arterially with a buffered glucose solution (Collin's solution) at 4°C; the addition of mannitol or citrate produces a hypertonic solution with greater stability and improved efficacy
5. The kidney is then placed on ice and kept cold by surface cooling; good renal function is achieved with this technique provided the initial warm ischaemia time is less than 5 minutes and transplantation occurs within 48 hours
6. Renal preservation is not required for kidneys from living related donors

Recipient operation
1. Heterotopic renal allotransplantation, implanting the graft retroperitoneally in either the right or left iliac fossa, is universally performed for the following reasons:
   a. No need to remove patient's own kidneys unless cause of refractory hypertension or a source of sepsis
   b. Implantation into this site is technically easier than into the normal anatomical position

c. Graft is superficial and easily accessible for biopsy and further surgery if required
2. An extra-peritoneal approach through an oblique muscle cutting incision in the iliac fossa exposes the iliac vessels at the pelvic brim
3. Left kidney is placed in right iliac fossa and vice versa
4. Renal vein is anastomosed end-to-side to the external or common iliac vein
5. Renal artery is anastomosed end-to-side to the external iliac artery or end-to-end with the divided internal iliac artery
6. Ureter is implanted into the bladder via a submucosal tunnel to prevent vesico-ureteric reflux

Complications

Immunological
1. Hyperacute rejection
   a. May be seen within the first few minutes of vascularising the transplanted kidney but can occur at any time within the first 48 hours
   b. Occurs in the presence of ABO blood group incompatibility and if the recipient has pre-existing cytotoxic antibodies to the major HLA antigens of the donor
   c. Characteristic histological features include polymorphonuclear infiltration, arteriolar and capillary thrombosis and interstitial haemorrhage
   d. The patient is typically unwell with a pyrexia and often rigors
   e. No satisfactory treatment exists and the transplant is normally removed
2. Accelerated rejection
   a. Occurs between the second and fifth post-operative days
   b. A severe systemic illness is accompanied by progressive oliguria and tender enlargement of the renal allograft
   c. Early treatment with intra-venous methylprednisolone is essential
   d. If the histological features include interstitial oedema, interstitial haemorrhage and vascular thrombosis the prognosis is poor
3. Acute rejection
   a. May occur any time between 5 days and 3 months following transplantation but is most commonly seen in the second and third weeks
   b. Reduced urine output follows swelling of the transplant and a variable systemic reaction; serum creatinine rises and creatinine clearance falls
   c. The classical feature on histological examination of renal biopsies is mononuclear cell infiltration

    d. Fibrinoid necrosis of the arteriolar walls may also be seen and is thought to indicate antibody mediated rejection

    e. Prompt treatment with methylprednisolone frequently restores renal function

4. Chronic rejection

    a. Occurs any time after 3 months and is associated with a gradual deterioration in renal function

    b. Hypertension and proteinuria are often seen

    c. Histological changes include interstitial fibrosis, intimal arterial fibrosis and glomerular hyalinisation

    d. Treatment with additional immunosuppresive agents has little beneficial effect

Non-immunological

1. Acute tubular necrosis

    a. Usually caused by an excessively long warm ischaemic time or prolonged hypotension in a cadaver donor

    b. Rarely seen in living-related grafts as total ischaemic time is very short

    c. Haemodialysis may be required in the oliguric phase

    d. Careful control of fluid and electrolyte balance is required in the diuretic phase

2. Renal artery and vein thrombosis

3. Ureteric obstruction

    a. May be caused by twisting or kinking of the ureter

    b. Intra-luminal blood clot or an ischaemic stricture are other causes

4. Urinary fistula

    a. Normally occurs in the first 6 weeks

    b. Is due primarily to ischaemia of the lower end of the transplanted ureter

5. Lymphocele

    a. Usually presents within the first 6 months of transplantation

    b. Usually due to failure to ligate lymphatics around the iliac vessels

    c. May cause obstruction to the ureter or iliac vein

6. Renal artery stenosis

    a. May occur at or distal to the arterial anastomosis and lead to hypertension and impaired graft function

    b. Onset may be delayed up to several years after transplantation

    c. Vascular reconstruction is technically difficult and percutaneous transluminal angioplasty may be preferred

7. Urinary tract infection

    a. Uraemia and immunosuppressive therapy predispose to infection

    b. Indwelling urethral or ureteric catheters specifically encourage urinary infection

Results

1. Graft survival (%)

	1 year	3 years	5 years
Living related donor	90–95	85–90	80–85
Cadaveric donor	70–85	60–75	50–70

2. Patient survival (%)

	1 year	3 years	5 years
Living related donor	95–98	90–95	85–90
Cadaveric donor	95	85–90	80–85

3. 90% of patients are rehabilitated to a normal life following successful transplantation
4. Patient survival exceeds graft survival by up to 50% as haemodialysis is used following graft rejection and prior to further transplantation
5. Various factors affect graft and patient survival
   a. Source of graft
      (i) Grafts from living related donors survive better than those from unrelated cadavers
      (ii) Grafts between HLA antigen identical siblings survive longer than those between non-identical siblings or parent and child
   b. Matching of HLA-antigens
      (i) Matching for HLA A, B and C antigens can improve long-term graft survival by up to 10%
      (ii) Matching for HLA DR antigens promotes graft survival even in the absence of HLA A, B and C compatibility
   c. Blood transfusion
      (i) Patients given blood transfusions before receiving a transplant show significantly better graft survival than non-transfused patients
      (ii) Donor-specific blood transfusions in living-related renal transplants have improved graft survival to over 95% at 1 year in one haplotype matched donor-recipient pairs
   d. Age of recipient
      (i) The best results of graft and patient survival are obtained in children aged 10–15 years
      (ii) Gradually reducing figures are achieved with increasing age over 45 years

FURTHER READING

Chisholm G D 1983 Renal transplantation (1). Hosp Update 9: 905–917
Chisholm G D 1983 Renal transplantation (2). Hosp Update 9: 961–975

Keowm P A, Stiller C B 1986 Kidney transplantation. Surg Clin N Am
    66: 517–540
Marshall V 1982 Organ preservation. In: Morris P J (ed) Clinical Surgery
    International Vol 3 Tissue Transplantation. Churchill Livingstone,
    Edinburgh pp 40–59
Morris P J 1982 Renal transplantation. In: Morris P J (ed) Clinical Surgery
    International Vol 3 Tissue Transplantation. Churchill Livingstone,
    Edinburgh pp 95–114
Morris P J 1985 Transplantation – the present position. In: Taylor I (ed)
    Progress in Surgery Vol 1. Churchill Livingstone, Edinburgh pp 133–146

LIVER TRANSPLANTATION

More than 1000 orthotopic liver allotransplants have been carried
out since the first operation was performed in 1963. Earlier
procedures were associated with a high mortality but later
refinements in operative technique and more effective
immunosuppressive regimens have improved both short and long
term results. Improved patient selection and earlier grafting of
patients with liver failure have also increased survival.

Indications
1. Cirrhosis
    a. Primary biliary cirrhosis
    b. Post-necrotic cirrhosis
    c. Cryptogenic cirrhosis
    d. Secondary biliary cirrhosis
2. Chronic active hepatitis
3. Subacute hepatic necrosis
4. Sclerosing cholangitis
5. Biliary atresia
6. Budd–Chiari syndrome
7. Inborn errors of metabolism
    a. α_1-antitrypsin deficiency
    b. Galactosaemia
    c. Wilson's disease
8. Primary liver tumours
    a. Hepatocellular carcinoma
    b. Cholangiocarcinoma

Contra-indications
1. Active infection
2. Age >50 years
3. Portal vein thrombosis
4. Primary extrahepatic malignancy
    More than half of all patients receiving liver transplants for
    hepatic metastases from a primary extra-hepatic malignancy
    develop recurrent tumour within 12 months
5. Metastatic hepato-biliary malignancy

6. Alcoholic cirrhosis
   Patients are unreliable at taking immunosuppressive therapy
   and attending for regular follow-up
7. Hepatitis-B surface antigenaemia
   A relative contraindication there being a risk of recurrent
   disease in the transplanted liver and significant hazards to staff
   and other patients

Operative technique

Donor operation
1. The donor must be ABO compatible with the recipient
2. Liver function tests must be within normal limits and the donor
   must be hepatitis-B surface antigen negative
3. A bilateral subcostal incision is made with upward extension to
   the xiphisternum
4. Following mobilisation of the liver, cannulae are inserted into
   the aorta, inferior vena cava and superior mesenteric vein
5. The liver is cooled in situ by perfusion with Hartmann's
   solution at 4°C followed by plasma protein fraction
6. Following removal of the liver, bile is removed from the gall
   bladder and bile ducts by perfusion to prevent damage to the
   biliary epithelium by bile salts

Recipient operation
1. Through a bilateral subcostal incision the liver is mobilised
   prior to trial cross-clamping of the inferior vena cava
2. If this is poorly tolerated partial cardio-pulmonary bypass via
   the right femoral artery and vein is commenced
3. The diseased liver is excised with a segment of inferior vena
   cava
4. The proximal end of the inferior vena cava attached to the
   hepatic graft is anastomosed to the recipient's supra-hepatic
   inferior vena cava
5. The portal veins of the donor and recipient are anastomosed
   end-to-end
6. Distal end of the donor inferior vena cava is anastomosed to
   the recipient's inferior vena cava following perfusion of the
   portal vein with warm plasma protein fraction
7. Donor coeliac artery is anastomosed to the recipient's hepatic
   artery
8. Donor and recipient common bile ducts are anastomosed end-
   to-end; as an alternative the donor gall bladder can be used as
   a conduit between the donor and recipient bile ducts

Complications

Immunological

1. Rejection
   a. Usually occurs between the third and fourth post-operative weeks but some degree of rejection is seen in most patients within the second post-operative week
   b. Characterised by tender hepatomegaly, jaundice and fever
   c. Diagnosed by a rise in serum bilirubin, alkaline phosphatase and liver transaminases and confirmed by percutaneous needle biopsy of the liver
   d. Treated with high doses of corticosteroids, usually methylprednisolone

Non-immunological

1. Vascular thromboses leading to graft infarction
2. Post-operative haemorrhage
3. Biliary anastomotic leakage
4. Biliary obstruction by inspissated sludge derived from slough of biliary epithelium
5. Septic cholangitis

Results

These have improved dramatically since the routine use of cyclosporin

1. Graft survival (%)

1 year	3 years	5 years
80	70	30

2. Patient survival is generally equivalent to graft survival, few recipients receiving more than one liver transplant
3. More than 50% of patients accepted for liver transplantation die before a suitable donor becomes available
4. 85% of patients surviving more than 6 months after liver transplantation return to school or work

FURTHER READING

Calne R Y 1982 Liver transplantation. In: Morris P J (ed) Clinical Surgery International Vol 3 Tissue Transplantation. Churchill Livingstone, Edinburgh pp 115–124

Calne R Y 1982 Liver transplantation. Hosp Update 8: 1203–1218

Kirby R M, McMaster P, Clements D et al 1987 Orthotopic liver transplantation: postoperative complications and their management. Br J Surg 74: 3–11

Van Thiel D H, Schade R R, Starzl T E 1985 Liver transplantation: after 20 years of experience the procedure has come of age. Curr Con Gastroenterol 2: 11–15

Williams R, Calne R Y, Rolles K, Polson R J 1985 Current results with orthotopic liver grafting in Cambridge/King's College Hospital series. Br Med J 290: 49–52

CARDIAC TRANSPLANTATION

Orthotopic cardiac allotransplantation was first performed in 1967 and the results improved considerably following the introduction of cyclosporin in 1980. More recently combined heart-lung transplantation has become feasible.

Indications

Cardiac transplantation is indicated in advanced cardiac disease with severe functional disability that is not amenable to conventional medical or surgical treatment and where the patient's prognosis is limited to a few months. The main conditions necessitating cardiac transplantation are:
1. Idiopathic cardiomyopathy
2. Severe valvular heart disease
3. Post-infarction ventricular aneurysm
4. Congenital heart disease
5. Coronary artery disease
6. Myocardial tumours

Combined heart/lung transplantation is now considered in cases of severe primary pulmonary hypertension and selected cases of Eisenmenger's syndrome.

Contra-indications
1. Active infection
2. Advanced age (>55–60 years)
3. Elevated pulmonary vascular resistance (>6 Wood units)
4. Insulin-dependent diabetes mellitus
5. Recent pulmonary infarction
6. Psychiatric disease
7. Severe hepatic or renal dysfunction
8. Disseminated malignant disease

Operative technique

Donor operation
1. Through a median sternotomy incision the donor heart is examined to exclude significant coronary artery disease
2. Following heparinisation and under venous inflow occlusion the aorta is cross-clamped
3. Aortic root is perfused with cold cardioplegic solution which arrests the heart in diastole
4. Heart is excised and after further washing in cold saline is placed in a sterile plastic bag containing cardioplegic solution at 4°C

Recipient operation
1. Median sternotomy is performed and the patient placed on cardio-pulmonary bypass
2. Heart is excised dividing the aorta and pulmonary artery immediately distal to their respective valves and leaving the posterior walls of the left and right atria in situ
3. After any necessary trimming the atrial cuffs of the donor heart are sutured to corresponding atrial remnants of the recipient's heart
4. The aortic and pulmonary anastomoses are then completed and following successful defibrillation cardio-pulmonary bypass is discontinued

Complications

Immunological
1. Acute rejection
   a. Usually occurs between the 8th and 12th post-operative week
   b. Characterised by cardiomegaly, pericardial effusion and reduced QRS voltages on ECG
   c. Diagnosed by serial trans-jugular endomyocardial biopsies performed at weekly intervals for the first six post-operative weeks and thereafter at less frequent intervals
   d. Treated by increasing oral prednisolone or giving intravenous methylprednisolone or anti-thymocyte globulin
2. Chronic rejection
   a. Occurs after the first three post-operative months
   b. Associated with accelerated atherosclerosis throughout the donor coronary arteries and is the most important cause of death in those patients surviving more than 1 year

Non-immunological
1. Pulmonary hypertension
2. Infections
   a. These are most commonly pulmonary and account for more than 50% of all deaths following cardiac transplantation
   b. Prompt diagnosis and aggressive anti-microbial therapy are required in cardiac transplant patients who are more immunosuppressed than those with renal or hepatic transplants
   c. Routine screening for chest infections includes regular chest radiography and sputum culture

Results
1. Graft survival (%)

1 year	3 years	5 years
75–80	50–70	40–60

2. Patient survival is generally equivalent to graft survival
   a. In the past few recipients received more than one cardiac allograft
   b. More recently, in a significant number of patients a second transplant has been thought to be feasible
3. Almost all patients accepted for transplantation and for whom no suitable donor is found fail to survive for 1 year
4. 80–90% of surviving cardiac transplant patients return to full activity and most resume active employment

FURTHER READING

Jamieson S W, Stinson E B, Shumway N E 1982 Cardiac transplantation. In: Morris P J (ed) Clinical Surgery International Vol 3 Tissue Transplantation. Churchill Livingstone, Edinburgh pp 147–160
English T A H 1982 Cardiac transplantation. Hosp Update 8: 1447–1454
McGregor C G A 1987 Current state of heart transplantation. Br J Hosp Med 37: 310–318

PANCREATIC TRANSPLANTATION

Pancreatic transplantation is indicated in insulin-dependent diabetics with severe renal impairment, who also suffer other major complications of diabetes mellitus. The procedure is therefore usually combined with renal allografting. A whole organ or segmental pancreatic graft is most commonly used although attempts have been made to transplant pancreatic islets by infusing them into the portal vein.

Surgical technique

Donor operation
1. Methylprednisolone and aprotinin (Trasylol) are given intra-venously immediately prior to the start of the donor operation
2. Both kidneys are first harvested in a routine manner
3. A distal segmental pancreatic graft comprises the body and tail of the pancreas and is mobilised by transection of the neck of the pancreas
4. The splenic artery is identified at its origin from the coeliac axis and the splenic vein where it drains into the portal vein
5. With a cannula in the coeliac axis the graft is perfused via the splenic artery using cold hypertonic citrate solution
6. The spleen is removed by careful ligation of the splenic vessels at its hilum
7. A pancreatico-duodenal graft is vascularised by the coeliac axis and superior mesenteric artery, venous drainage being provided by the portal vein

Recipient operation
1. Standard renal transplantation is performed, the graft usually being placed in the left iliac fossa
2. A segmental pancreatic allograft is placed in the contralateral iliac fossa
3. The donor coeliac axis or splenic artery is anastomosed end-to-side to the recipient external iliac artery
4. Donor splenic vein is anastomosed end-to-side to the external iliac vein
5. Pancreatic duct is either injected with a polyisoprene or neoprene latex polymer or drained into the ipsilateral ureter or a jejunal Roux loop
6. A pancreatico-duodenal transplant can be anastomosed to a jejunal Roux loop but better results have been obtained with drainage into the urinary bladder

Complications

Immunological
Rejection is suggested by an increase in fasting and post-prandial blood sugar levels but these changes tend to occur when most of the graft has already been destroyed. It can be confirmed by angiography or radio-isotope scintigraphy. The uptake of indium labelled platelets shows some promise as an earlier indicator of graft rejection. If the exocrine secretions are drained into the bladder pancreatic enzyme levels can be used to monitor graft function.

Non-immunological
1. Exocrine pancreatic fistula
2. Vascular thrombosis
3. Pancreatic atrophy and fibrosis

Results
1. Patient survival
   a. The operative mortality of segmental pancreatic transplantation is quite high largely because the procedure is performed on severely debilitated, uraemic, diabetic patients
   b. Mortality rates of up to 75% were initially recorded but these have now fallen to approximately 33%
2. Graft survival
   a. Graft survival rates have been disappointing with only 30% surviving longer than one year
   b. Whole organ grafts drained into the urinary bladder promise to give improved success rates
   c. The results of pancreatic transplantation in the absence of a renal graft are so poor that the two procedures are nearly always performed simultaneously

FURTHER READING

McMaster P 1983 Pancreas transplants. Hosp Update 9: 369–374
Groth C G, Gunnarsson R, Lundgren G, Ostman J 1982 Pancreatic
   transplantation. In: Morris P J (ed) Clinical Surgery International Vol 3
   Tissue Transplantation. Churchill Livingstone, Edinburgh pp 125–146
Sutherland D E R, Kendall D, Goetz F C, Najarian J S 1986 Pancreas
   transplantation. Surg Clin N Am 66: 557–582

Endocrine surgery

PHAEOCHROMOCYTOMA (CHROMAFFINOMA)

Introduction
1. 90% of phaeochromocytomas are benign, the remainder showing varying degrees of malignancy
2. 10% of phaeochromocytomas in adults and 25% in children are outside the adrenal glands. Extra-adrenal locations include the organ of Zuckerkandl, para-aortic and para-vertebral regions and the urinary bladder
3. 5–10% of adrenal tumours in adults and 25% in children are bilateral
4. In about 10% of cases phaeochromocytomas are associated with other neuroendocrine abnormalities including neurofibromatosis, medullary carcinoma of the thyroid gland, parathyroid adenomas and multiple endocrine adenomatosis (Type II MEA syndrome)
5. The clinical features associated with a phaeochromocytoma are due to increased concentrations of circulating catecholamines secreted by the tumour
6. Phaeochromocytomas account for 0.1% of all cases of hypertension

Clinical features
1. Hypertension is persistent in half of all cases and paroxsymal in the remainder
2. Paroxsyms of hypertension may be associated with headache, palpitations, flushing, pallor, hyperhidrosis, nausea, vomiting, abdominal pain and acute anxiety states
3. Paroxsymal symptoms often occur spontaneously but are also precipitated by several factors including exertion, emotional upsets and various drugs including anaesthetic agents
4. Impaired glucose tolerance, hyperglycaemia and overt diabetes mellitus

Diagnosis
1. Total plasma cathecholamine level >1.0 μg/l
2. Urinary adrenaline excretion >20 μg/24 h
3. Urinary noradrenaline excretion >70 μg/24 h
4. Urinary 4-hydroxy 3-methoxy mandelic acid (HMMA) excretion >35 μmol/24 h
5. Clonidine suppression test
6. Pentolinium suppression test
7. Provocative tests using histamine, tyramine or glucagon may be dangerous producing uncontrollable hypertension and are therefore no longer routinely used

Localisation
The presence of a high noradrenaline:adrenaline ratio suggests a phaeochromocytoma in an extra-adrenal site.
1. Plain abdominal radiography
2. Intravenous urography
3. Ultrasonography
4. Scintigraphy using ^{131}I meta-iodobenzylguanidine (MIBG)
5. Aortography and selective adrenal arteriography may provoke hypertension and should only be performed in patients who are fully prepared as for surgery (see below).
6. Vena caval catheterisation and selective venous catheterisation with sampling and measurement of plasma catecholamine levels
7. Computed tomography

Pre-operative preparation
1. Adrenergic receptor blockade
   a. α-blockers reduce the increased vasoconstrictor tone and reduce the systemic blood pressure
   b. Phenoxybenzamine 0.5 mg/kg body weight is given by intravenous infusion over 2 hours each day for three days
   c. Phentolamine is infused intra-venously for rapid control of severe hypertension
   d. β-blockers such as propanolol 40 mg 8-hourly are used if a marked tachycardia or other arrhythmias are present
   e. Propranolol must not be given before the α-blockade has been established
2. Restoration of circulating blood volume
   a. Reduction of vasoconstrictor tone produces an increased circulatory capacity
   b. Restoration of the blood volume is achieved with appropriate intravenous fluids

Surgical management
1. An anterior abdominal approach allows both adrenal glands to be examined

2. The lumbar sympathetic chain and the pelvis are also examined for synchronous tumours
3. Large adrenal tumours may require a thoraco-abdominal approach
4. An attempt should be made to occlude the venous drainage of the tumour prior to its manipulation: excessive handling of the tumour may cause release of large amounts of catecholamines with dramatic changes in blood pressure
5. Intra-operative hypertensive crises are treated with nitroprusside
6. Following removal of the tumour a profound fall in blood pressure may occur due to a marked reduction in vascular tone
7. Large volumes of intra-venous fluids may be required to restore the patient's circulating blood volume

FURTHER READING

Hunt T K, Roizen M F, Tyrrell J B, Biglieri E G 1984 Current achievements and challenges in adrenal surgery. Br J Surg 71: 983–985
McDougal W S 1984 Surgery of the adrenal. In: Dudley H A F, Pories W J, Carter D C (eds) Operative Surgery: Urology. 4th Edition. Butterworths, London, pp 13–20

CUSHING'S SYNDROME

Aetiology
1. Iatrogenic
   Therapeutic adminstration of supraphysiological doses of cortico-steroids or adreno-corticotrophic hormone (ACTH) is the commonest cause of Cushing's syndrome
2. Pathological
   a. Pituitary-dependent bilateral adrenocortical hyperplasia (Cushing's disease) (75%)
      Basophil pituitary adenoma secretes excessive amounts of ACTH
   b. Adreno-cortical tumours (20%)
      Autonomous adrenal adenomas are usually single and are more common than carcinomas which may be bilateral
   c. Ectopic ACTH syndrome (5%)
      This is due to inappropriate ACTH secretion by benign or malignant tumours of non-endocrine origin, e.g. oat-cell carcinoma of lung

Clinical features
1. Male:female ratio is 1:4
2. Peak age incidence is 35–50 years
3. Patients usually present with diabetes mellitus or hypertension

4. Other clinical features include:
   a. Truncal and facial obesity
   b. Purple striae
   c. Excessive bruising
   d. Osteoporosis and pathological fractures
   e. Muscle weakness
   f. Hirsutism
   g. Polyuria
   h. Psychoses

Diagnosis
1. Plasma cortisol levels.
   While morning cortisol levels may be normal, patients with Cushing's disease show loss of the normal diurnal variation in plasma cortisol levels
2. 24-hour urinary cortisol excretion.
   Values greater than 1000 nmol in males and 776 nmol in females support a diagnosis of Cushing's syndrome
3. Insulin tolerance test.
   Patients with Cushing's disease fail to increase their circulating cortisol levels in response to hypoglycaemia
4. Low-dose dexamethasone suppresion test.
   Failure to suppress the morning cortisol level to below 170 nmol/l confirms the diagnosis of Cushing's syndrome

Determination of cause
1. Radio-immunoassay of plasma ACTH
   a. If ACTH is either not detectable or very low the patient has an autonomous adrenal tumour
   b. Plasma ACTH levels are raised in Cushing's disease and very high in cases of ectopic ACTH syndrome
2. Metyrapone test.
   A large increase in plasma ACTH and urinary cortico-steroids following metyrapone confirms a diagnosis of Cushing's disease
3. High-dose dexamethasone suppression test.
   A 50% suppression of plasma and urinary cortico-steroids occurs in Cushing's disease but not in other causes of Cushing's syndrome

Localisation of unilateral adrenal disease
1. Plain abdominal radiography.
   Adrenal calcification may indicate an underlying tumour, usually a carcinoma
2. Intravenous urography (IVU) with tomography.
   Inferior displacement of a kidney or distortion of its calyces indicates the presence of an adrenal tumour

3. Scintigraphy.
   ^{131}I-iodo-cholesterol is taken up by benign tumours
4. Ultrasound scan
5. Computed tomography
6. Selective venous catheterisation
   a. Adrenal venous blood is sampled and its plasma cortisol level measured
   b. Retrograde venography may show a tumour circulation
7. Arteriography

Treatment
Bilateral adrenalectomy in unprepared patients with Cushing's syndrome is associated with a 5% mortality. All patients with Cushing's syndrome undergoing surgical treatment should be prepared with metyrapone which inhibits the 11β-hydroxylase enzyme essential for steroid biosynthesis.
1. Cushing's disease
   a. Bilateral adrenalectomy
      (i) An anterior trans-peritoneal approach allows access to both adrenal glands
      (ii) Separate posterior extra-peritoneal approaches provide an alternative surgical route and minimise the complications of wound sepsis and impaired healing in those patients with advanced Cushing's disease
      (iii) Pituitary irradiation should always be given following adrenalectomy to prevent hyperpigmentation (Nelson's syndrome)
      (iv) Maintenance hydrocortisone and fludrocortisone are required to prevent hypoadrenalism
   b. Pituitary ablation
      (i) Indicated if a hypophyseal tumour has been demonstrated
      (ii) Hypophysectomy via a trans-sphenoidal or trans-frontal route
      (iii) External beam pituitary irradiation
      (iv) Intra-pituitary ^{90}Y yttrium implants
2. Adrenal tumours
   a. Unilateral adrenalectomy for adenomas
   b. Bilateral adrenalectomy may be required for synchronous adrenal carcinomas
   c. Post-operative radiotherapy is given to the bed of malignant tumours to prevent local recurrence
   d. Ortho, p'DDD and aminoglutethimide which both inhibit the early stages of steroid biosynthesis are used to treat metastatic disease
3. Ectopic ACTH syndrome
   a. Source of ACTH secretion is removed after metyrapone preparation

b. Long-term treatment with metyrapone or aminoglutethimide is given for inoperable tumours and supplemented by replacement steroid therapy

FURTHER READING

McDougall W S 1984 Surgery of the adrenal. In: Dudley H A F, Pories W J, Carter D C (eds) Operative Surgery: Urology. 4th Edition. Butterworths, London pp 13–20
Hunt T K, Roizen M F, Tyrrell J B, Biglieri E G 1984 Current achievements and challenges in adrenal surgery. Br J Surg 71: 983–985
Jeffcoate W J 1988 Treating Cushing's disease. Br Med J 296: 227–228
Nabarro J 1986 Transsphenoidal surgery for Cushing's syndrome. J R Soc Med 79: 253–254
Falbusch R, Buchfelder M, Muller O A 1986 Transsphenoidal surgery for Cushing's syndrome. J R Soc Med 79: 262–269

THYROTOXICOSIS

Aetiology
1. Graves' disease (primary thyrotoxicosis)
2. Secondary thyrotoxicosis
   a. Toxic multinodular goitre
   b. Solitary toxic (hot) thyroid nodule

Clinical features
1. Graves' disease is an auto-immune disorder which usually occurs in young adult females and is associated with the presence of a diffuse smooth goitre often with a bruit
2. Secondary thyrotoxicosis tends to occur in older patients
3. General features of thyrotoxicosis which are related to an accelerated metabolic rate and mediated by the sympathetic nervous system include:
   a. weight loss despite increased appetite
   b. heat intolerance
   c. tachycardia
   d. hyperhidrosis
   e. tremor
   f. anxiety states
4. Ophthalmic signs are often seen in Graves' diseases but rarely in cases of secondary thyrotoxicosis:
   a. lid retraction
   b. lid lag
   c. chemosis
   d. exophthalmos
   e. periorbital oedema
   f. ophthalmoplegia

5. Less common features of thyrotoxicosis include proximal myopathy, pretibial myxoedema and thyroid acropathy
6. The cardiac manifestations of thyrotoxicosis are more likely to occur in elderly patients
   a. angina pectoris
   b. atrial fibrillation
   c. congestive cardiac failure

Treatment

1. Carbimazole
   a. An initial dose of 15 mg tds is reduced to 10 mg tds when the patient becomes euthyroid
   b. Maintenance thyroxine may be required to prevent hypothyroidism
   c. Propranolol or an alternative β-adrenergic receptor blocking agent may be required in the first 2–4 weeks of anti-thyroid drug therapy to provide adequate symptomatic control in severely thyrotoxic patients
   d. If used in attempt to treat primary thyroxicosis definitively carbimazole must be continued for at least 1 year
   e. Side effects include skin rashes and agranulocytosis
   f. Spontaneous remission often occurs when carbimazole therapy is discontinued but over 50% of patients relapse within 2 years and almost 75% of patients have relapsed after 5 years
   g. Relapse following carbimazole therapy is more common in patients who initially present with severe thyrotoxicosis
2. Subtotal thyroidectomy
   a. Indications for operative treatment are:
      (i) relapse after a prolonged course of carbimazole
      (ii) poor response to anti-thyroid drugs
      (iii) poor compliance, drug intolerance or severe side effects
      (iv) large goitre
      (v) severe thyrotoxicosis in young patients
      (vi) patient's preference for surgical treatment
   b. Many surgeons now consider that surgical treatment is the preferred method of treatment of primary hyperthyroidism once the patient has been rendered euthyroid with carbimazole or the symptoms and signs of thyrotoxicosis controlled by β-blockers
   c. Lugol's iodine may be given for 7–10 days pre-operatively
   d. Complications of thyroidectomy include:
      (i) recurrent laryngeal nerve palsy (1%)
      (ii) external laryngeal nerve palsy (1–5%)
      (iii) hypoparathyroidism (1–2%)
      (iv) recurrent hyperthyroidism (1–5%)
      (v) hypothyroidism (20%)

Half of those patients who become hypothyroid do so within 6 months of surgery but in some cases it is transient. Hypothyroidism is more common in patients with lymphocytic infiltration of the thyroid gland and those with antibodies to thyroid microsomes and thyroglobulin.

3. Radio-active iodine (^{131}I)
   a. Usually reserved for patients over 40 years of age and its use is contraindicated in children
   b. Most useful in elderly patients and those unfit for surgery or with recurrent thyrotoxicosis following subtotal thyroidectomy
   c. Standard therapeutic dose (5–10 mCi) produces hypothyroidism in 20% of patients at 1 year and 50% after 10 years, necessitating the lifelong use of replacement thyroxine therapy; in addition up to 25% of patients may suffer recurrent hyperthyroidism within 1 year of treatment
   d. Ablative dose (20–30 mCi) will rapidly control hyperthyroidism in all patients with minimal risk of relapse; the incidence of hypothyroidism is much greater than with a standard therapeutic dose of radio-active iodine being 60% at 1 year and 95% at 5 years

4. Treatment of ophthalmic complications (thyrotoxic ophthalmopathy)
   a. Mild complications: treatment is designed to prevent damage to the exposed cornea
      (i) Methyl cellulose eye drops
      (ii) 5% guanethidine eye drops
      (iii) Protective glasses
      (iv) Lateral tarsorrhaphy
   b. severe progressive congestive ophthalmopathy (malignant exophthalmos):
      (i) High dose cortico-steroids – prednisolone 60 mg/day or dexamethasone 20 mg/day – to prevent optic nerve damage
      (ii) Azathioprine
      (iii) Surgical decompression of the orbit
      (iv) Total thyroidectomy, pituitary ablation and orbital irradiation

FURTHER READING

Cusick E L, Krukowski Z H, Matheson N A 1987 Outcome of surgery for Graves' disease re-examined. Br J Surg 74: 780–783
Harada T, Shimaoka K, Mimura T, Ho K 1987 Current treatment of Graves' disease. Surg Clin N Am 67: 299–314
Reid D J 1987 Hyperthyroidism and hypothyroidism complicating the treatment of thyrotoxicosis. Br J Surg 74: 1060–1062

Sheldon J, Reid D J 1986 Thyrotoxicosis: changing trends in treatment. Ann R Coll Surg Eng 68: 283–285
Russell R C G 1986 Thyroidectomy. Br J Hosp Med 35: 327–303

SOLITARY THYROID NODULES

Pathology

1. Thyroid nodules diagnosed clinically as solitary are found in 50% of cases to be multiple either at surgical exploration or on histological examination of the excised thyroid tissue
2. A true solitary thyroid nodule is one of the following:
   a. Adenomatous (hypertrophic or colloid) nodule with secondary changes such as haemorrhage, necrosis, cystic degeneration, fibrosis or calcification (60%)
   b. Adenoma (30%)
   c. Carcinoma (10%)
   d. Localised area of chronic lymphocytic (Hashimoto's) thyroiditis (<1%)
3. Solitary thyroid nodules are more common in women than men
4. The risk of malignancy in a solitary thyroid nodule is 20–30% in males and may be as high as 40% in children and adolescents of either sex
5. Most patients with solitary thyroid nodules even those with functioning adenomas are euthyroid
6. Features of hyperthyroidism suggest the presence of a toxic adenoma

Investigation

As only a minority of solitary thyroid nodules are malignant it has been suggested that surgery can be avoided in many patients by selection on the basis of various investigations.

1. Radio-isotope scintigraphy
   a. 99m technetium pertechnetate is used to establish the functional status of thyroid nodules in relation to the rest of the thyroid gland
   b. Should not be performed in children or pregnant women
   c. Nodules may be classified as cold (no uptake), neutral or warm (normal uptake) or hot (increased uptake)
   d. The majority of thyroid nodules are cold; most are adenomatous nodules, cysts or adenomas but carcinoma accounts for 15–20% of all cold nodules
   e. Isotope uptake by a thyroid nodule does not exclude a carcinoma, usually well-differentiated, which is found in approximately 5% of warm nodules
   f. Less than 5% of thyroid nodules are hot: a hot nodule is very rarely malignant

2. Ultrasonography
   a. An easily performed non-invasive investigation without dangers which can be performed in children and pregnant women and repeated on several occasions
   b. As sound waves are reflected by bone a retro-sternal thyroid cannot be examined
   c. Modern ultrasound machines with a high resolution can detect lesions greater than 2 mm in diameter
   d. Although ultrasound accurately distinguishes solid from cystic lesions it cannot determine their underlying pathology
   e. Both benign and malignant tumours can undergo varying degrees of cystic degeneration
   f. Patients with cystic lesions may be suitable for aspiration and cytological examination of the fluid obtained
   g. A residual swelling or recurrence of the cyst following aspiration suggests the presence of a carcinoma
   h. Injection of sclerosant agents such as sodium tetradecyl sulphate (STD) may help to prevent recurrence of simple thyroid cysts
   i. Adenomas, carcinomas and adenomatous nodules may all present as solid lesions on ultrasound but have no distinguishing features
3. Percutaneous large needle biopsy
   a. A Tru-cut or similar needle is used to remove a core of tissue under local anaesthetic
   b. Tumour cells may possible be disseminated along the needle track
   c. Other complications include haematoma formation and transient recurrent laryngeal nerve palsy
   d. Small lesions may be difficult or even impossible to biopsy
   e. As with any blind biopsy technique there is always a potential problem of sampling error
4. Fine needle aspiration cytology
   a. A popular technique in Scandinavian countries for many years
   b. A fine needle is used to obtain a cellular sample of the thyroid swelling
   c. Subsequent cytological examination requires considerable expertise
   d. In experienced hands 80–90% accuracy is possible although a distinction between adenomatous nodule, follicular adenoma and carcinoma is not usually feasible
   e. Differentiation between Hashimoto's thyroiditis and lypmhoma may also be difficult
   f. Negative cytological examination of a clinically suspicious lesion should always be followed by surgical exploration

Surgical exploration and histological examination

1. In many cases a pre-operative diagnosis is not available and the lobe of the thyroid gland containing the nodule must be excised and subjected to histological examination
2. Excised surgical specimens should be examined immediately by an experienced pathologist
3. Histological examination of frozen sections of thyroid tumours is often useful but the surgeon must appreciate its difficulties
4. Papillary carcinomas are easily recognised
5. Poorly differentiated carcinomas invading normal thyroid tissue are easily identified although they may be difficult to differentiate from a lymphoma
6. In well-differentiated carcinomas the appearance of follicular cells may be indistinguishable from those seen in benign conditions and the diagnosis of carcinoma then rests on the identification of vascular or capsular invasion
7. Histological evidence of invasion may not be detectable on the few frozen sections examined histologically at the time of surgery
8. Under these circumstances thyroid lobectomy with removal of the adjacent isthmus should be performed; if subsequent paraffin section reveal the presence of a follicular carcinoma adequate surgical treatment will have been performed

FURTHER READING

Matheson N A 1986 The diagnosis of thyroid swellings. In: Russell R C G (ed) Recent Advances in Surgery Vol 12 Churchill Livingstone, Edinburgh pp 179–197
Lennquist S 1987 The thyroid nodule: diagnosis and surgical treatment. Surg Clin N Am 67: 213–232
Peake R L 1987 Clinical evaluation of thyroid tumors. In: Thawley S E, Panje W R, Batsakis J G, Lindberg R D (eds) Comprehensive Management of Head and Neck Tumors W B Saunders, Philadelphia pp 1580–1598
Sykes D 1981 The solitary thyroid nodule. Br J Surg 68: 510–512
Werk E E, Vernon B M, Gonzalez J J, Ungaro P C, McCoy R C 1984 Cancer in thyroid nodules: a community hospital survey. Arch Int Med 144: 474–476

THYROID TUMOURS

Benign tumours

1. Papillary adenoma
   a. A benign thyroid tumour showing a papillary pattern is extremely rare
   b. It is safer to regard all papillary tumours as malignant; those which appear histologically benign with no evidence of capsular, lymphatic or blood vessel invasion are best classified as well differentiated papillary carcinomas

2. Follicular adenoma
   a. Presence of a well defined capsule allows differentiation from a colloid nodule
   b. May be classified as embryonal, fetal or simple depending on the degrees of differentiation and follicle formation and the size of the follicles
   c. Macrofollicular (colloid) adenoma contains an excessive amount of colloid within large distended follicles
   d. Hurthle (oxyphil) adenoma contains large acidophylic granular cells, shows minimal signs of follicle formation and contains very little colloid
   e. Degenerative changes within follicular adenomas include cyst formation, haemorrhage, fibrosis and calcification
   f. Usually slow growing and often functional but only rarely do follicular adenomas become autonomous to produce a 'toxic adenoma'
   g. Not currently thought to be pre-malignant
3. Teratoma
   a. A rare tumour seen exclusively in young infants and invariably benign
   b. The presence of calcification is diagnostic

Malignant tumours

Malignant thyroid tumours exhibit a wide range of malignant potential. They account for 0.5% of all deaths from malignant disease but occult thyroid carcinoma is found in up to 10% of patients at post-mortem examination. In general thyroid carcinoma has a relatively good prognosis in young patients but this deteriorates over the age of 40 years especially in males.

Many thyroid carcinomas present as a solitary thyroid nodule. Others present as diffuse or nodular enlargements of the thyroid gland and occasionally with lymph node or distant metastases. The presence of a hard fixed mass, hoarse voice or Horner's syndrome signify extra-capsular spread and a poorer prognosis.

Patients under 30 years of age tend to have papillary carcinomas while follicular carcinoma is rare in this age group.

The extent of the surgical resection employed in the treatment of differentiated thyroid carcinomas remains controversial. The risks of total thyroidectomy are significantly greater than those of subtotal resection but in experienced hands the increased risk is small. In total thyroidectomy both recurrent laryngeal nerves are exposed to the risk of injury and damage or removal of the parathyroid glands may lead to permanent hypoparathyroidism with its associated morbidity. Each case must be carefully assessed and the risks of damage to these structures weighed against the risk of recurrent malignant disease. The commonly accepted surgical management of papillary and follicular carcinomas based on the degree of thyroid involvement and the presence of metastatic disease is outlined below.

1. Papillary carcinoma (55–60%)
   a. Commonest malignant thyroid tumour usually occurring in young adult females with a peak incidence in the third and fourth decades
   b. 30–50% of cases have multicentric disease within the thyroid gland
   c. Usually a slow growing tumour which metastasises via lymphatics to regional lymph nodes in approximately half of all cases; distant metastases are extremely rare and only 2% of patients die as a direct result of their malignant disease
   d. In older age groups papillary carcinoma runs a more aggressive course with 15–20% dying of the disease
   e. May present with cervical lymph node metastases from an occult primary lesion
   f. For apparently unilateral disease total thyroid lobectomy is performed on the side of the lesion with subtotal lobectomy on the contralateral side
   g. Total thyroidectomy is performed when both lobes show gross involvement by tumour or there is evidence of extensive cervical or mediastinal lymph node disease or distant metastases
   h. Adjacent pre-tracheal and para-tracheal lymph nodes are excised at the time of thyroidectomy if possible
   i. Patients with impalpable cervical lymph nodes require no further treatment; prophylactic cervical lymph node dissection and external beam radiotherapy are of no proven value
   j. Recurrent disease in the cervical lymph nodes is generally treated by local excision which may be repeated as required
   k. Modified radical cervical lymph node dissection in which the internal jugular vein, spinal accessory nerve and sterno-cleidomastoid muscle are preserved may be useful in preventing further recurrent disease but it does not affect prognosis
   l. Radical cervical lymph node dissection in patients with palpable cervical lymph nodes is rarely performed as it too does not affect the long-term prognosis and may cause considerable morbidity; the substernal and mediastinal lymph nodes which are important routes of tumour dissemination are not removed in this dissection
   m. Suppressive doses of thyroxine are given to all patients regardless of whether total thyroidectomy has been performed as papillary tumours are TSH-dependent and thyroxine reduces the incidence of recurrence
   n. Prognosis is related to the extent of local disease at the time of presentation; intra-thyroid papillary carcinoma has

a 90% 10-year survival rate compared with 50% 10-year survival for patients with tumours that extend beyond the capsule of the thyroid

o. Involvement of cervical lymph nodes does not affect overall prognosis

2. Follicular carcinoma (15–25%)

   a. Tends to occur in older age groups with a peak incidence in the fifth and sixth decades

   b. Commonly metastasises to bone and lungs but lymphatic spread is unusual

   c. Although often well encapsulated the tumour is characterised by the presence of vascular invasion

   d. Primary surgical treatment of small tumours should consist of total thyroid lobectomy with excision of the thyroid isthmus

   e. Patients with larger tumours and those with prominent capsular or vascular invasion are treated by total thyroidectomy

   f. If disseminated disease is present total thyroidectomy is performed to allow the metastases to be more effectively treated with radioactive iodine

   g. All patients should receive a suppressive dose of thyroxine

   h. As lymphatic spread is extremely rare cervical lymph node dissection is not routinely performed

   i. Most follicular carcinomas take up iodine and radio-active iodine is commonly used in the treatment of metastatic disease; TSH stimulation may be useful

   j. Prognosis is less favourable than for papillary tumours and is related to the histological grade of the tumour and its degree of vascular invasion

   k. Patients with tumours showing marked invasion have a 60% 5-year survival rate compared with over 90% in those with only slight invasion

3. Anaplastic (undifferentiated) carcinoma (10%)

   a. Rapidly growing and usually lethal tumour seen in elderly patients

   b. Extension of the tumour across the thyroid isthmus to the contralateral lobe is common

   c. Extensive extra-capsular invasion with infiltration of the adjacent structures of the neck is commonly seen

   d. Lymphatic and haematogenous metastases occur readily

   e. Total thyroidectomy is rarely feasible but should be attempted if there is no evidence of extra-capsular invasion or distant metastases

   f. Prophylactic local radiotherapy is given following thyroidectomy to prevent reccurrent disease

   g. Where total thyroidectomy is not possible central resection is performed: the isthmus is excised along with the medial part of each lobe to free the trachea and provide material for histological examination

h. Post-operative radiotherapy provides a useful response in many cases but pre-operative treatment is of no value

i. Chemotherapy is used if there is a poor response to radiotherapy

j. Prognosis is very poor with a 20% 1-year survival

k. Death is usually due to uncontrollable tumour growth within the neck

4. Medullary carcinoma ('solid adenocarcinoma with amyloid stroma') (5–7%)

a. Often a slow-growing tumour which tends to occur in older age groups

b. 15% of cases are familial being inherited via an autosomal dominant trait

c. Derived from para-follicular (C) cells and may secrete calcitonin

d. Characteristic histological features include the presence of small round or spindle-shaped cells lying in a hyaline stroma which gives a positive staining reaction for amyloid

e. May be associated with phaeochromocytoma and multiple neuromas (Type 2 multiple endocrine neoplasia, MEN II)

f. Usually multicentric within the thyroid gland

g. Invades extra-thyroid tissues and has a great propensity to invade lymphatics and metastasise to cervical lymph nodes

h. Invasion of blood vessels is usually evident and distant metastases especially of the lungs and liver are often seen

i Total thyroidectomy should be performed and any palpable lymph nodes excised

j. Plasma calcitonin levels can be used to determine the presence of residual or recurrent disease

k. Prognosis is determind by the grade of malignancy and the lymph node status at presentation

l. 80% 10-year survival for node-negative cases; 40% 10-year survival for node-positive cases

5. Lymphoma

a. The thyroid is often involved in cases of disemminated disease but occasionally a lymphoma is localised to the thyroid gland

b. Primary malignant lymphoma of the thyroid occurs mainly in elderly women

c. Localised lymphoma may arise in previously existing auto-immune thyroiditis but the risk does not justify routine total thyroidectomy in all cases of Hashimoto's disease: adequate suppressive therapy with thyroxine reduces the risk of malignant change

d. Wide central resection is followed by radiotherapy as the tumour is usually very radiosensitive

6. Sarcoma
   a. A rare tumour which tends to occur in elderly patients
   b. Various histological types are seen
7. Secondary tumours
   a. Usually occur as a feature of extensive disseminated disease
      so that the nature of the thyroid mass is readily suspected
   b. Common primary tumours metastasising to the thyroid
      gland include malignant melanoma, hypernephroma and
      breast and bronchial carcinomas

Thyroid cancer in children
1. 80% of thyroid tumours in children are associated with
   previous irradiation, usually in infancy with a latent period of
   about 10 years
2. Radiation induced thyroid cancers do not behave more
   aggressively than those arising spontaneously
3. Most tumours are well-differentiated papillary carcinomas
   which are associated with cervical lymph node or pulmonary
   metastases at the time of presentation
4. Even in the presence of disseminated disease papillary thyroid
   tumours run a slow clinical course in childhood

FURTHER READING

Beahrs O H 1984 Surgical treatment for thyroid cancer. Br J Surg
    71: 976–979
Beahrs O H 1987 Controversy in the management of tumours of the thyroid
    and parathyroid glands. In: Thawley S E, Panje W R, Batsakis J G,
    Lindberg R G (eds) Comprehensive Management of Head and Neck
    Tumours. W B Saunders, Philadelphia pp 1679–1684
Block M A 1987 Surgical therapy of thyroid tumors. In: Thawley S E, Panje
    W R, Batsakis J G, Lindberg R D (eds) Comprehensive Management of
    Head and Neck Tumors. W B Saunders Philadelphia pp 1616–1634
Brunt L M, Wells S A 1987 Advances in the diagnosis and treatment of
    medullary thyroid cancer. Surg Clin N Am 67: 263–280
Palmer B V, Harmer C L, Shaw H J 1984 Calcitonin and carcino-embryonic
    antigen in the follow-up of patients with medullary carcinoma of the
    thyroid. Br J Surg 71: 101–104
Poston G J, Lynn J A 1986 Endocrine tumours of the neck. In: Bloom H J G,
    Hanham I W F, Shaw H J (eds) Head and Neck Oncology pp 171–187.
    Raven Press, New York pp 171–187
Schwartz A E, Friedman E W 1987 Preservation of the parathyroid glands in
    total thyroidectomy. Surg Gynecol Obstet 165: 327–332
Shah J P 1986 Differentiated thyroid cancer. In: Bloom H J G, Hanham
    I W F, Shaw H J (eds) Head and Neck Oncology Raven Press, New York
    pp 207–214
Vickery A L, Wang C-A, Walker A M 1987 Treatment of intrathyroidal
    papillary carcinoma of the thyroid. Cancer 60: 2587–2595
Wade J S H 1983 The management of malignant thyroid tumours. Br J Surg
    70: 253–255

Werner B, Abele J, Alveryd A et al 1984 Multimodal therapy in anaplastic giant cell thyroid carcinoma. World J Surg 8: 64–70

HYPERPARATHYROIDISM

Classification
1. Primary hyperparathyroidism
   a. Single parathyroid adenoma (85%)
   b. Multiple parathyroid adenomas (5%)
   c. Diffuse hyperplasia of all parathyroid glands (10%)
   d. Parathyroid carcinoma (<1%)
   Primary hyperparathyroidism may be associated with multiple endocrine adenomatosis.
2. Secondary hyperparathyroidism.
   An increased secretion of parathormone is appropriate to the patient's low serum ionised calcium level
3. Tertiary hyperparathyroidism.
   Chronic hypocalcaemia especially due to renal failure leads to parathyroid hyperplasia. Secretion of parathormone by the hyperplastic tissue eventually becomes autonomous resulting in hypercalcaemia

Presentation
1. Incidental finding of hypercalcaemia on routine biochemical screening (Serum Multiple Analysis) (35%)
2. Urinary tract calculi and nephrocalcinosis (20%)
3. Metabolic bone disease (5%)
4. Polydipsia and polyuria
5. Peptic ulceration
6. Acute pancreatitis
7. Constitutional symptoms, e.g. lethargy, weight loss, anorexia
8. Psychiatric disorders, e.g. depression, neurosis, confusion dementia, psychosis
9. Gastro-intestinal symptoms, e.g. abdominal pain, nausea and vomiting, constipation
10. Musculo-skeletal symptoms, e.g. muscle weakness, aches and pains
11. Acute hypercalcaemic crisis characterised by dehydration, confusion or hypercalcaemic coma

Differential diagnosis of hypercalcaemia
Hyperparathyroidism is one of many causes of hypercalcaemia. It is not the commonest cause.
1. Malignant disease expecially breast and bronchial carcinoma and myelomatosis
2. Primary and tertiary hyperparathyroidism
3. Sarcoidosis
4. Milk-alkali syndrome

5. Vitamin D toxicity
6. Paget's disease
7. Adrenal insufficiency
8. Thyrotoxicosis
9. Thiazide diuretics
10. Idiopathic hypercalcaemia of infancy (Elfin face syndrome)

Diagnosis of hyperparathyroidism

1. Exclude other obvious causes of hypercalcaemia
2. Persistent hypercalcaemia (corrected plasma calcium concentration > 2.55 mmol/l) on three consecutive venous blood samples taken whilst fasting in the presence of an inappropriate serum level of parathormone
3. Radiological features include generalised osteoporosis, subperiosteal bone resorption, bone cysts and loss of the dental lamina dura
4. Steroid suppression test will usually cause a fall in the serum calcium level in all cases of hypercalcaemia not due to hyperparathyroidism

Pre-operative parathyroid gland localisation

This is usually reserved for those patients with persistent or recurrent hypercalcaemia following previous exploration of the neck in whom anatomical distortion and scar tissue may render intra-operative parathyroid gland localisation quite difficult.

1. Selective venous catheterisation with multiple venous blood sampling and parathormone assay is a technically difficult procedure requiring a highly skilled operator; it accurately localises glands prior to initial surgery in about 80% of patients but its success is less in those undergoing reoperation
2. Double radio-isotope (technetium–thallium) subtraction scintigraphy can locate 80–90% of parathyroid adenomas prior to initial surgical exploration
3. Ultrasound scanning only reveals relatively large glands situated in the neck which would normally be easily apparent at surgery; glands situated behind the sternum, trachea or oesophagus are not visualised by ultrasound
4. Selective arteriography only localises 50% of abnormal glands and has several risks
5. Computed tomography is often useful in identifying certain ectopic glands especially those in the mediastinum but its overall accuracy is only 50%

As no technique is completely accurate they are often combined.

Surgical treatment

1. Parathyroid surgery should be a careful, systematic and bloodless exploration

2. The parathyroid glands usually lie symmetrically on the posterior surface of the thyroid gland and they are normally a dull orange or brown colour
3. The superior (IV) parathyroid glands are normally found adjacent to the inferior thyroid artery just after it has started to branch
4. The inferior parathyroid (III) glands are usually adjacent to the lower pole of the thyroid gland
5. Scrupulous haemostasis prevents discoloration of the tissues which may impair recognition of parathyroid tissue
6. All four parathyroid glands should be identified; identification can be aided by various techniques:
   a. Pre-operative intra-venous infusion of methylene blue (5 mg/kg body weight in 500 ml 5% dextrose infused over 1 hour immediately prior to surgery)
   b. Flotation test
   c. Biopsy and frozen section (cryostat) histological examination
7. 15% of parathyroid glands lie in one of several ectopic sites:
   a. adjacent to the superior thyroid vessels
   b. adjacent to the carotid sheath
   c. within the thymus
   d. within the thyroid gland
   e. behind the larynx, pharynx or oesophagus
   f. within the anterior or posterior mediastinum
   The thymus may have to be delivered into the neck and removed but exploration of the mediastinum via a median sternotomy is rarely required.
8. A single adenoma is excised; snip biopsy of the remaining parathyroid glands to exclude coincident hyperplasia may lead to hypocalcaemia
9. In parathyroid hyperplasia three glands are removed completely alongwith half the fourth gland. The residual tissue is marked with a black silk suture or metal clip in case re-exploration for recurrent hypercalcaemia is required. Auto-transplantation of the remaining parathyroid tissue into the muscles of the fore-arm, again marked with a silk suture, will avoid the need for further exploration of the neck in these circumstances. Transitory or permanent hypocalcaemia are recognised complications of this latter method

FURTHER READING

Bainbridge E T, Barnes A D 1983 Some changing aspects of primary hyperparathyroidism. Ann R Coll Surg Engl 65: 67–70
Barnes A D 1984 The changing face of parathyroid surgery. Ann R Coll Surg Engl 66: 77–80

Editorial 1986 Parathyroid gland localisation. Lancet ii: 726–727

Lavelle M A, Glover F N 1984 Parathyroidectomy. Br J Hosp Med 31: 204–208

Poston G J, Lynn J A 1986 Endocrine tumours of the neck. In: Bloom H J G, Hanham I W F, Shaw H J (eds) Head and Neck Oncology Raven Press, New York pp 171–187

Sherlock D J, Holl-Allen R J 1984 Intravital methylene blue staining of parathyroid glands and tumours. Ann R Coll Surg Engl 66: 396–398

Smith R 1984 Hypercalcaemia: presentation. Br J Hosp Med 31: 174–184

Thomas J M, Cranston D, Knox A J 1985 Hyperparathyroidism – patterns of presentation, symptoms and response to operation. Ann R Coll Surg Engl 67: 79–82

Wells S A, Leight G S, Farndon J R 1982 Transplantation of endocrine tissues. In: Morris P J (ed) Clinical Surgery International Vol 3: Tissue Transplantation Churchill Livingstone, Edinburgh pp 226–241

Young A E 1984 Localisation of parathyroid glands. Br J Hosp Med 31: 198–203

Young A E, Gaunt J I, Croft D N, Collins R E C, Wells C P, Coakley A J 1983 Location of parathyroid adenomas by thallium-201 and technetium-99m subtraction scanning. Br Med J 286: 1384–1386

CARCINOID TUMOURS AND THE CARCINOID SYNDROME

Carcinoid tumours

Carcinoid tumours (argentaffinomas) arise from the argentaffin cells which form part of the amine precursor uptake and decarboxylation (APUD) system. These cells which produce peptide hormones are found throughout the gastro-intestinal tract and are orginally of neural crest origin. Carcinoid tumours may also arise in the respiratory and biliary tracts and in the ovaries.

Sites of origin

Vermiform appendix	40%
Small intestine (mainly ileum)	20%
Large intestine (mainly rectum)	20%
Lung and bronchus	10%
Other sites, e.g. stomach, biliary tree, ovary	10%

1. Most carcinoid tumours of the appendix and rectum are benign and are usually incidental findings
2. Tumours at these sites greater than 2 cm in diameter have malignant potential
3. Colonic and jejuno-ileal carcinoids are often multiple and usually behave in a malignant fashion often presenting with massive regional lymph node and hepatic metastases
4. Even malignant carcinoid tumours are often slow growing
5. Patients with carcinoid tumours have an increased incidence of other tumours derived from APUD cells

Presentation
1. Incidental finding, approximately 0.5% of all surgically removed appendices contain a carcinoid tumour, usually near the tip of the appendix
2. Abdominal mass
3. Intestinal obstruction which is often due to intussusception
4. Gastro-intestinal haemorrhage
5. Bronchial obstruction which may lead to pneumonia or atelectasis
6. Carcinoid syndrome

Surgical treatment of primary carcinoid tumours
1. Appendix
   a. Standard appendicectomy if the tumour is less than 2 cm
   b. Larger tumours or those with vascular invasion, involvement of the mesoappendix or evidence of regional spread should be treated by radical right hemicolectomy
2. Small intestine and colon
   a. Segmental resection with removal of the regional lymph nodes
   b. Metastatic disease is not a contraindication to resection
3. Rectum
   a. Small asymptomatic tumours should be locally excised
   b. If greater than 2 cm a rectal carcinoid tumour should be treated by radical resection
4. Bronchial carcinoids are treated by pulmonary lobectomy or pneumonectomy as appropriate

Prognosis
This is related to the following factors:
1. Site of the primary tumour
2. Size of primary tumour
3. Extent of loco-regional spread
4. Presence of distant metastases

Typical 5-year survival rates:

Vermiform appendix	99%
Rectum	83%
Bronchus	67%
Colon	52%
Small intestine	54%

Carcinoid syndrome
1. Symptoms of the carcinoid syndrome are due to release of serotonin (5-hydroxy-tryptamine) and other hormonal peptides such as kallikrein into the systemic circulation
2. Malignant carcinoid tumours of the gastro-intestinal tract therefore only produce the carcinoid syndrome when metastases are present in the liver

3. In contrast bronchial and ovarian carcinoid tumours may produce the syndrome in the absence of hepatic metastases as their venous drainage is directly into the systemic circulation
4. Diagnosis is confirmed by elevated serum serotonin levels or increased urinary excretion of 5-hydroxyindole acetic acid (5-HIAA), the metabolite of serotonin

Clinical features
1. Hepatomegaly
2. Facial flusing often precipitated by exercise, emotion or alcohol
3. Cutaneous telangiectasia of the face
4. Bronchoconstriction
5. Episodic watery diarrhoea with noisy borborygmi
6. Right-sided heart failure due to fibrotic valvular disease, typically pulmonary stenosis and tricuspid regurgitation

Treatment
1. Anti-serotonin agents, e.g. methysergide, cyproheptadine, para-chlorophenylalanine may help control diarrhoea
2. Alpha-adrenergic blocking agents, e.g. phenoxybenzamine are used to control flushing attacks
3. Cytotoxic chemotherapy, e.g. 5-fluorouracil, streptozotocin
4. Hepatic arterial embolisation
5. Hepatic artery ligation
6. Enucleation of hepatic metastases
7. Hepatic resection
   a. Manipulation of metastases at operation may cause massive release of vasoactive mediators leading to severe bronchoconstriction and profound hypotension (carcinoid crisis)
   b. Pharmacological antagonists should always be available during hepatic surgery

FURTHER READING

Ahlman H 1986 Midgut carcinoid tumours. In: Nyhus L M (ed) Surgery Annual 1986. Appleton-Century-Crofts, Norwalk, Connecticut
Dawes L, Schulte W J, Condon R E 1984 Carcinoid tumours. Arch Surg 119: 375–378
Moertel C G, Weiland L H, Nagorney D M, Dockerty M B 1987 Carcinoid tumour of the appendix: treatment and prognosis. New Eng J Med 317: 1699–1701
Welch J P, Malt R A 1977 Management of carcinoid tumours of the gastrointestinal tract. Surg Gynecol Obstet 145: 223–227
Godwin J D 1975 Carcinoid tumours. Cancer 36: 560–569

ZOLLINGER–ELLISON SYNDROME

Pathogenesis

1. Massive hypersecretion of gastric acid due to high plasma levels of gastrin produced usually by a pancreatic islet cell tumour
2. 60% of gastrinomas are malignant although many are slow growing
3. 50% of patients have multicentric disease or metastases within the pancreas
4. More than half of all patients with the Zollinger–Ellison syndrome have hepatic metastases at the time of surgery
5. Gastrinomas are occassionally found in ectopic sites such as the duodenal submucosa

Clinical features

The diagnosis of Zollinger–Ellison syndrome should be suspected in the following circumstances:

1. Peptic ulcer refractory to adequate medical treatment
2. Duodenal ulceration in very young or very eldery patients
3. Early recurrent peptic ulceration following an adequate surgical procedure
4. Large gastric mucosal folds with excessive fluid in an unobstructed stomach
5. Fulminating ulcer diathesis with multiple peptic ulcers throughout the duodenum and even in the proximal jejunum
6. Peptic ulceration associated with persistent diarrhoea or Type 1 multiple endocrine neoplasia (MEN I)

Diagnosis

Hypergastrinaemia is seen in any condition associated with gastric acid hyposecretion eg gastric carcinoma, atrophic gastritis, pernicious anaemia. To diagnose Zollinger–Ellison syndrome it is necessary to demonstrate excessive gastric acid secretion associated with hypergastrinaemia. The following tests are used to confirm the diagnosis of Zollinger–Ellison syndrome:

1. Basal acid output (BOA) > 15 mEq/h
2. 12-hour overnight gastric secretion > 1 litre
3. 12-hour overnight gastric acid secretion > 100 mEq
4. Basal plasma gastrin level > 100 pg/ml
5. Ratio of maximal to basal acid output (MAO:BAO) < 3
6. Provocation tests
   a. Calcium or secretin provocation tests are accompanied by a marked increase in serum gastrin levels to at least twice the basal level
   b. Meal provocation test produces no increase in serum gastrin levels in patients with Zollinger–Ellison syndrome

Localisation of gastrinoma

1. Ultrasonography usually fails to reveal the pancreatic tumour as it is often less than 3 mm in diameter
2. Computed tomography may also have insufficient resolution to identify very small tumours
3. Arteriography is often of little use as gastrinomas may be relatively avascular
4. Direct selective portal venous catheterisation via percutaneous trans-hepatic route allows cannulation of several veins draining the pancreas: assay of venous blood for gastrin allows the tumour bearing segment of the pancreas to be identified

Treatment

1. H$_2$-receptor antagonists
   a. Medical treatment with H$_2$-receptor antagonists effectively reduces gastric acid hypersecretion in most patients and provides useful temporary symptomatic relief
   b. They do not have the morbidity and mortality associated with a major surgical procedure
   c. Ranitidine (Zantac) is more effective than cimetidine (Tagamet) in controlling acid secretion and has fewer side effects; it is the treatment of choice in patients who refuse or are unfit for surgery
2. Surgery
   a. Surgical treatment is dependent on pre-operative tumour localisation and the findings at laparotomy
   b. A solitary pancreatic tumour without obvious spread is treated by local excision or segmental pancreatic resection if it is situated in the tail
   c. Total pancreatectomy should be avoided as subsequent recurrence may require total gastrectomy with serious nutritional consequences
   d. If metastases are present at the initial laparotomy total gastrectomy is performed in those patients not adequately controlled with ranitidine
3. Chemotherapy
   a. Various chemotherapeutic agents have been used in patients with unresectable metastatic disease but their effects are unpredictable
   b. Streptozotocin, 5-fluorouracil and adriamycin are reported to be of benefit in controlling the growth and spread of tumour in some patients

FURTHER READING

Deveney C W, Deveney K E 1987 Zollinger–Ellison syndrome (Gastrinoma). Current diagnosis and treatment. Surg Clin N Am 67: 411–422

Kaplan E L, Michelassi F 1986 Endocrine tumours of the pancreas and their clinical syndromes. In: Nyhus L M (ed) Surgery Annual 1986. Appleton-Century-Crofts, Norwalk, Connecticut pp 181–223

Modlin I M, Brennan M F 1984 The diagnosis and management of gastrinoma. Surg Gynecol Obstet 158: 97–104

Thompson N W, Eckhauser F E 1984 Malignant islet-cell tumours of the pancreas. World J Surg 8: 940–951

WATERY DIARRHOEA SYNDROME

Introduction
A rare syndrome characterised by profuse watery diarrhoea and usually associated with a non-beta islet cell tumour of the pancreas secreting excessive quantities of vasoactive intestinal polypeptide (VIP).

Synonyms include:
1. Pancreatic cholera
2. WDHA syndrome (Watery Diarrhoea, Hypokalaemia and Achlorhydria)
3. Verner–Morrison syndrome

Clinical features
1. Profuse watery diarrhoea
   a. This may be constant or intermittent
   b. It is not related to meals and in some cases may be explosive
   c. Faecal volumes up to 10 litres per day have been recorded but the average output is half this amount
   d. Dehydration and hypovolaemic shock may occur
2. Hypokalaemia due to severe loss of potassium in the faecal fluid
3. Achlorhydria or hypochlorhydria
4. Metabolic acidosis
5. Hypercalcaemia is present in half of all cases and is not usually caused by parathyroid disease
6. Hyperglycaemia or impaired tolerance to a glucose load occurs in over 50% of patients
7. Uraemia

Pathogenesis
Most patients with WDHA have markedly raised serum levels of vasoactive intestinal polypeptide (VIP). This hormone inhibits gastric acid secretion, stimulates alkaline secretion by the pancreas and impairs small intestinal water and ion resorption. The colon is unable to absorb the vastly increased amounts of water and electrolytes passing through the ileo-caecal valve.

1. Pancreatic lesions are found in 90% of cases of WDHA syndrome
   a. 80% of patients have islet cell tumours of which more than half are malignant and readily metastasise
   b. Islet cell hyperplasia is seen in the remaining 20%
2. Extra-pancreatic tumours account for the remaining 10% of patients
   a. ganglioneuroma
   b. phaeochromocytoma
   c. neuroblastoma
   d. bronchogenic carcinoma

Differential diagnosis
1. Laxative abuse
2. Large intestinal villous adenoma
3. Parasitic infestation
4. Bacterial infections
5. Coeliac disease
6. Inflammatory bowel disease
7. Zollinger–Ellison syndrome
8. Carcinoid syndrome
9. Medullary carcinoma of thyroid

Diagnosis
Serum vasoactive intestinal polypeptide level >2000 pg/ml

Localisation of vipoma
1. Elevated serum pancreatic polypeptide (PP) concentration indicates the presence of a tumour in the pancreas
2. Percutaneous trans-hepatic catheterisation of pancreatic veins with venous sampling and assay of VIP levels
3. Computed tomographic scanning of the lungs and retroperitoneum to exclude extrapancreatic tumours

Treatment
1. Correction of fluid and electrolyte imbalance
2. Steroids (prednisolone 40 mg/day) provide symptomatic control of diarrhoea in 50% of patients
3. Indomethacin inhibits prostaglandin synthesis and control of the diarrhoea may be improved
4. Somatostatin infusion
5. Surgery
   a. 80% of benign pancreatic VIPomas are located in the body or tail and are readily amenable to local excision
   b. Malignant tumours should be resected where possible
   c. If curative resection is not feasible debulking operations will often palliate the symptoms

d. Subtotal (80%) distal pancreatectomy is reserved for patients with islet cell hyperplasia

6. Chemotherapy

a. Streptozotocin or cyclophosphamide combined with 5-fluorouracil have been used with success in patients with disseminated malignant disease

b. Decreased levels of VIP accompany subjective improvements in patients responding to chemotherapy

FURTHER READING

Kaplan E L, Michelassi F 1986 Endocrine tumours of the pancreas and their clinical syndromes. In: Nyhus L M (ed) Surgery Annual 1986 Appleton-Century-Crofts, Norwalk, Connecticut pp 181–223

Thompson N W, Eckhauser F E 1984 Malignant islet-cell tumours of the pancreas. World J Surg 8: 940–951

Orthopaedic surgery

FRACTURES

Principles of management
1. Reduction of fracture
2. Maintenance of reduction
   a. Skeletal or skin traction
   b. External splintage (plaster of Paris, external fixators)
   c. Internal fixation
3. Rehabilitation

Indications for internal fixation
1. Failure to achieve or maintain adequate reduction by external means (e.g. fracture of femoral neck)
2. Fracture involving a joint surface which requires very accurate anatomical reduction (e.g. Bennett's fracture, ankle fractures)
3. Multiple long bone fractures in one limb
4. Pathological fractures
5. Need for early mobilisation in elderly patients
6. Neurovascular complications

Complications of internal fixation
1. Infection
2. Delayed union
3. Non-union
4. Fracture of implant due to metal fatigue

Complications of fracture healing
1. Mal-union is union of a fracture with an angular or rotational deformity or unacceptable shortening
2. Delayed union represents a delay in the normal time for fracture healing to have occurred; there is no radiological evidence of non-union
3. Non-union is characterised radiologically by sclerosis at the bone ends; bony union will not occur without further surgery.
   a. Hypertrophic non-union is characterised by proliferative new bone around the fracture ends to give the typical 'elephant boot' appearance radiologically

b. Atrophic non-union is characterised by atrophied bone ends which have a spiked appearance

Causes of malunion, delayed union and non-union
1. Poor blood supply to the bone fragments, e.g. fractures of the distal third of the tibia, and waist of the scaphoid
2. Double fracture of a long bone
3. Wide separation of the fracture surfaces, e.g. loss of bone substance in gunshot fractures, excessive muscle retraction of bone fragments, excessive traction leading to over-distraction
4. Severe compound fracture with major soft tissue damage
5. Infection
6. Interposition of soft tissue such as muscle and periosteum between the fracture surfaces

Treatment of non-union
1. Hypertrophic non-unions respond well to bone grafting procedures with or without external fixation
2. Atrophic non-unions are more difficult to treat as bone grafting is frequently unsuccessful.
   a. There is some evidence that electrical stimulation of the fracture ends promotes healing but it is not conclusive.
   b. Vascularised bone grafts may be indicated. Refer to Page 255
   c. In some cases there is no alternative to amputation

Compound fractures
All compound fractures of bones should be treated as surgical emergencies.
1. Immediate treatment
   a. Resuscitation with intra-venous fluids and blood transfusion. Refer to Page 212
   b. Analgesics
   c. Systemic antibiotics should include broad-spectrum agents with specific activity against *Staphylococcus aureus*
   d. Anti-tetanus prophylaxis
   e. External splintage
2. Surgical treatment
   a. Surgical debdridement must be performed within 6 hours of the injury
   b. Thorough wound toilet is followed by excision of all dead tissue
   c. Adjacent tissues are examined to ensure that structures such as tendons and nerves are intact
   d. Fasciotomy may be required to prevent impairment of the distal circulation
   e. Primary wound closure is ideal but may not be possible due to wound tension

   f. In such cases the wound is either left open or a split-thickness skin graft applied

   g. Internal fixation is contraindicated

   h. The fracture is often best controlled by the use of an external fixator

FURTHER READING

Wilson J N (ed) 1976 Watson Jones Fractures and Joint Injuries (5th edn). Churchill Livingstone, Edinburgh

KNEE JOINT INJURIES

Collateral ligament injuries

These occur as a direct result of a valgus or varus injury to the knee joint. They may occur in isolation or in conjunction with a cruciate ligament or meniscal injury. The treatment is dependent on the severity of the injury.

1. Simple sprain
   a. All the ligament fibres remain in continuity
   b. Treatment includes analgesics and non-steroidal anti-inflammatory drugs
   c. Physiotherapy and hydrotherapy are also very useful

2. Partial tear
   a. Only a portion of the ligament fibres remain in continuity
   b. More pain and bruising are present than after a simple sprain but there is no clinical or radiological evidence of joint instability
   c. A plaster cylinder is applied for 6 weeks followed by a course of physiotherapy

3. Complete tear
   a. Complete disruption of the ligament fibres occurs often with an associated capsular tear
   b. The knee joint is clinically unstable
   c. Diagnosis is confirmed by examination under anaesthetic and stress radiographs
   d. The injury may be associated with an internal derangement of the knee joint
   e. Following a complete tear the ligament fibres retract and the defect is filled by scar tissue if repair is not undertaken

    f. Conservative treatment often causes the ligament to heal with some laxity resulting in an unstable joint: such treatment which involves immobilisation in a plaster cylinder for 6 weeks may be appropriate in some elderly patients

    g. Immediate surgical repair is normally indicated in younger patients

Anterior cruciate ligament injuries

1. Anterior cruciate injury is the commonest cause of haemarthrosis in the adult
2. Anterior cruciate ligament is taut in full flexion and internal rotation of the tibia
3. It may be ruptured in isolation by forced flexion and internal rotation of the tibia or in combination with collateral ligament injury
4. The diagnosis is suggested by the presence of a haemarthrosis with a positive anterior draw sign and a positive Lachman sign
5. A radiograph of the injured knee may show an avulsed fragment of bone detached from the site of insertion of the ruptured ligament
6. Arthroscopy identifies the degree of injury and the site of rupture; it also allows lavage of the haemarthrosis
7. If the ligament has been avulsed from bone at either end surgical repair is indicated especially in young patients
8. Repair of the anterior cruciate ruptured at its mid part usually gives poor results
9. Long-term complication of anterior cruciate rupture is antero-lateral knee joint instability resulting in a positive jerk or pivot shift test

Posterior cruciate ligament injury

1. Posterior cruciate ligament may be damaged by a blow on the anterior aspect of the flexed knee or in combination with collateral ligament injuries
2. Positive posterior draw sign confirms the diagnosis
3. Treatment is conservative unless a bone fragment at the site of insertion has been avulsed

Meniscal injuries

1. The injury is caused by a rotatory force on the weight bearing flexed knee
2. Various types of tear are recognised:
    a. Bucket handle tear
    b. Anterior horn tag tear
    c. Posterior horn tag tear
    d. Peripheral detachment
    e. Horizontal cleavage tear

3. Symptoms include the following:
   a. Pain
   b. Swelling
   c. Feeling of joint instability
   d. Mechanical locking of knee joint
4. Physical signs include the following
   a. Joint effusion
   b. Quadriceps wasting
   c. Joint line tenderness
   d. Extension block (locked knee)
   e. Positive McMurray test
5. Investigations
   a. Plain radiographs of the knee joint are taken to exclude other pathology
   b. Arthrography may yield a positive diagnosis but accuracy is dependent on interpretation by a skilled radiologist
   c. Arthroscopy is now increasingly used to confirm a clinical diagnosis
6. Surgical management
   a. Complete removal of the torn meniscus is usually avoided if at all possible
   b. Arthroscopic meniscectomy has the great advantage over open operation of rapid rehabilitation and return to work
   c. The torn part of the meniscus is excised and the major portion of the cartilage remains in situ to minimise the development of degenerative changes within the knee joint

Causes of a locked knee
1. Loose intra-articular body
   a. Osteophyte formation secondary to osteoarthritis
   b. Osteochondral fracture
   c. Osteochondritis dissecans
   d. Synovial osteochondromatosis
2. Meniscal tear

FURTHER READING

Dandy D J 1982 Arthroscopic surgery of the knee. Br J Hosp Med 27: 360–365
Insall J N 1984 Surgery of the knee. Churchill Livingstone, Edinburgh

OSTEOARTHRITIS

Any synovial joint may be affected by 'wear and tear' degenerative arthritis but it is more common in the load bearing joints such as the hip and knee. Osteoarthritis is more common in the Western World than in developing countries.

Aetiology
1. Primary osteoarthritis has no known cause
2. Secondary osteoarthritis
   a. Congenital abnormalities, e.g. congenital dislocation of the hip joint
   b. Trauma – fractures involving a joint surface
   c. Infection, e.g. pyogenic or tuberculous arthritis
   d. Connective tissue disorders, e.g. rheumatoid arthritis

Radiological features
1. Loss of joint space
2. Sclerosis of joint margins
3. Bone cyst formation
4. Osteophytes

Principles of management
1. Conservative treatment
   a. Weight reduction
   b. Walking aids, e.g. walking stick or frame
   c. Analgesics
   d. Non-steroidal anti-inflammatory drugs
   e. Physiotherapy including hydrotherapy
   f. Aids in the house supplied by occupational therapist
2. Surgical treatment
   a. Total replacement arthroplasty, e.g. total hip replacement, total knee replacement
   b. Osteotomy, e.g. upper femoral, upper tibial osteotomy
   c. Arthrodesis, e.g. ankle, subtalar and mid-tarsal joints
   d. Excision arthroplasty, e.g. Keller's arthroplasty for hallux rigidus

Surgical treatment of osteoarthritis of hip joint
1. Total replacement arthroplasty
   a. Is now the most common surgical procedure for osteoarthritis of the hip
   b. The high density polyethylene acetabular component and the titanium or cobalt chrome femoral component are fixed in situ with methylacrylic cement
   c. Complications include infection, loosening and recurrent dislocation
   d. Refer to Page 209
2. Upper femoral osteotomy
   a. Suitable for younger patients without femoral head collapse and with a reasonable range of abduction and adduction of the hip joint
   b. Either a varus or valgus osteotomy may be performed
   c. The principle is to realign the weight bearing area of the hip joint

3. Arthrodesis
  a. Now rarely accepted by patients
  b. Occasionally still appropriate for severe osteoarthritis secondary to trauma in young male patients

Surgical treatment of osteoarthritis of knee joint
1. Upper tibial osteotomy
  a. Valgus osteotomy of the upper tibia is performed for medial compartment disease
  b. The principle is to realign the load bearing surface of the knee joint
  c. For best results the degenerative changes should be confined to the medial compartment, the joint should flex to at least 90° and the patient should be under 65 years
2. Arthrodesis of knee joint
  a. The principle is to convert a stiff, painful joint into a totally stiff painless joint
  b. The ipsilateral hip joint should show no signs of degenerative disease
3. Total knee replacement
  a. It has been considerably more difficult to design prostheses for knee replacement than for hip replacement because of the inherent instability of the knee joint and the design of replacements for the cruciate ligaments
  b. Modern knee replacements are very much improved on the earlier models
  c. Emphasis is now on re-surfacing prostheses which allow normal movements at the knee joint and maintain stability
  d. Refer to Page 210

FURTHER READING

Engh C A, Babyn J D 1985 Biological fixation in total hip arthroplasty. Slack

ARTHROPLASTY
Arthroplasty is the surgical refashioning of a joint designed to relieve pain and/or improve joint mobility.

Types of arthroplasty
1. Excision arthroplasty – both joint surfaces are excised and not replaced, e.g. Girdlestone's operation, Keller's operation
2. Interposition arthroplasty – insertion of a liner or spacer into the joint, e.g. Helal arthroplasty
3. Hemiarthroplasty – excision and replacement of one joint surface, e.g. Austin Moore hemiarthroplasty
4. Total replacement arthroplasty – excision and replacement of both joint surfaces, e.g. total hip replacement

Features of an ideal replacement arthroplasty
1. Provides complete relief of pain
2. Produces an adequate range of movement without compromising joint stability
3. Is capable of bearing the loads required
4. Has a low coefficient of friction
5. Has a low rate of wear
6. Made from materials which are tissue compatible in the formed or wear product state
7. In the event of component failure or complications the design of the prosthesis should allow for revision surgery

Materials used for joint replacement
1. Ultra-high molecular weight polyethylene (UHMWPE)
   a. Used as a weight-bearing surface against metal with the following characteristics:
      (i) Decreased friction
      (ii) Decreased metal wear products
      (iii) Decreased wear resistance as compared to metal on metal
   b. Most common material for the acetabular components of total hip replacements
2. Titanium
   a. A very strong alloy containing aluminium and vanadium
   b. Low incidence of allergic reaction and is therefore used in patients with a history of metal allergy
   c. Requires anodising to prevent excessive wear
   d. Expensive
   e. Most commonly used material for the femoral component of total hip replacements; is also used in a number of the tibial components of total knee replacements
3. Cobalt-chrome alloys
   a. Several types are available containing differing amounts of nickel, molybdenum and titanium
   b. Very corrosion resistant
   c. Manufactured by casting
   d. High tensile strength but quite expensive
4. Silicone elastomers
   a. A very flexible material which is quite inert
   b. Poor load-bearing characteristics
   c. Ideal for use as a spacer in the finger joints and for replacing the first metatarso-phalangeal joint (Helal spacer)
5. Polymethylmethacrylate
   a. Cold-polymerising plastic compound used as a cement to secure prosthetic components of a conventional joint replacement
   b. Antibiotics may be added to the cement to reduce the incidence of infection especially in revisional surgery

Complications of replacement arthroplasties

1. Infection
    a. Incidence of infection can be reduced by:
        (i) prophylactic systemic antibiotics
        (ii) antibiotic-loaded cement
        (iii) laminar air flow ventilation in operating theatres
        (iv) stringent aseptic technique
    b. Infection rate should be less than 0.5%
2. Mechanical loosening
    a. Breakdown of the bond between the bone and the cement results in loosening of the components and eventually loss of bone stock
    b. Incidence of loosening is decreased by improved cement techniques:
        (i) dry operative field
        (ii) lavage systems
        (iii) cement guns to introduce cement under pressure
        (iv) cement restrictors
    c. When loosening occurs early revision surgery is now advocated, the revision being performed before loss of bone stock occurs
    d. Morbidity and mortality of revision surgery are significantly higher and the long-term results poorer than those of first-time replacements
3. Component failure
    a. With some early designs and materials femoral stem fractures were seen
    b. With the introduction of better designs and improved materials, especially titanium, these problems are less commonly encountered
4. Metal sensitivity
    a. Thought to be the cause of mechanical loosening particularly in implants which contain nickel
    b. Factors other than metal sensitivity are probably more important
5. Dislocation
    a. Most commonly occurs with total hip replacements
    b. Recurrent dislocation is nearly always due to surgical error in implantation and orientation of the prosthesis

Individual joints

1. Hip joint
    a. Most commonly performed arthroplasty
    b. Hemi-replacement arthroplasty (e.g. Thompson's prosthesis) in which only the femoral head is replaced is most frequently performed for subcapital femoral neck fractures

   c. With conventional cemented total hip replacement arthroplasty emphasis is now on use of a straight stemmed femoral component with a high-density polyethylene acetabular component

   d. Acetabular component may be metal-backed to improve cement fixation

   e. Use of a large femoral stem allows the medullary canal to be filled with metal thereby reducing the thickness of the layer of bone cement

   f. Improved cement techniques have decreased the incidence of mechanical loosening but this remains a significant problem in younger patients

   g. Uncemented hip replacements aim to eliminate the problems of mechanical loosening especially in younger patients: two main types are now available:
      (i) Press fit prosthesis, e.g. Link prosthesis
      (ii) Porous coated prosthesis, e.g. Harris Galante prosthesis which allows for bone ingrowth into the prosthesis to occur

   h. Long term results of these prostheses are as yet unknown

   i. The principle of resurfacing replacements is to resurface the femoral head with minimal removal of bone

   j. The results of resurfacing replacements have so far been poor and the technique is not widely used

   k. Excision arthroplasty is most commonly used as a salvage procedure for failed total hip replacement arthroplasty especially if a prosthesis becomes infected

2. Knee joint
   a. Unconstrained resurfacing knee replacements (e.g. Insall Burstein prosthesis)
      (i) Allow for minimal bone resection and in the event of failure may be converted to a hinged prosthesis or an arthrodesis
      (ii) All normal movements can occur at the joint thus reducing the incidence of mechanical loosening
      (iii) Stability is dependent on the collateral ligaments
      (iv) Precise surgical technique is required for implantation of the prosthesis
      (v) Initial results are very encouraging

   b. Semi-constrained knee replacement (e.g. Attenborough prosthesis)
      (i) Loose links between the femoral and tibial components allow for inherent stability
      (ii) Once popular but now used less frequently

   c. Hinged knee replacement
      (i) Ease of insertion and rapid post-operative rehabilitation are the main advantages

      (ii) Allows for flexion and extension only; due to torsional stresses this type of replacement has a high rate of mechanical loosening

      (iii) Used in the treatment of severely incapacitated rheumatoid arthritic patients with many joints affected and who will therefore place low demands on the knee joint replacement

      (iv) Also used for revision knee surgery

  d. Unicompartmental knee replacements

      (i) introduced as an alternative to osteotomy when disease is confined to either the medial or lateral compartment of the knee joint

      (ii) Allows for minimal bone resection

      (iii) Long-term results are not yet available

3. Shoulder joint

  a. Replacement arthroplasty is used as an alternative to arthrodesis

  b. Main indication is relief of pain

  c. Total replacement arthroplasty may be indicated in patients with severe rheumatoid arthritis or avascular necrosis of the humeral head

  d. Problems have been encountered with fixation of the glenoid component but new prostheses are very much improved

  e. Design of the glenoid component should ideally prevent proximal migration of the humerus

  f. The most important factor governing the end result is good post-operative rehabilitation

  g. Scrupulous attention should be paid to repair of the rotator cuff

  h. Hemi-replacement arthroplasty in which only the humeral head is replaced may be indicated in patients with severe humeral neck fractures, such as four part fractures, and patients with avascular necrosis of the humeral head

4. Elbow joint

  a. Excision arthroplasty may produce useful function and pain relief in a severely diseased joint

  b. Hinged prosthetic total replacement arthroplasty does not have particularly good long-term results due to mechanical loosening

  c. Resurfacing of the humerus and olecranon is more encouraging

5. Finger joints

  a. Metacarpo-phalangeal joints may need to be replaced in cases of severe rheumatoid arthritis

  b. A hinged or elastomer spacer is used

  c. Correction of deformity, by tendon balancing or soft tissue release, prior to insertion of the implants is essential

    d. Pre-operative hand function must be carefully assessed
    e. Cosmetic appearance is not an indication for arthroplasty
    f. Arthroplasty of the proximal and distal interphalangeal joints is rarely indicated
6. Wrist joints
    a. Excision arthroplasty of individual carpal bones, e.g. trapezium for osteoarthritis of the first carpo-metacarpal joint
    b. Excision of individual bones and replacement of silastic spacer, e.g. scaphoid or lunate for avascular necrosis
    c. Excision of distal ulnar styloid for mal-united Colles' fracture or in combination with synovectomy for rheumatoid arthritis

FURTHER READING

Engh C A, Bobyn J D 1985 Biological fixation in total hip arthroplasty. C B Slack, Thoroughfare, New Jersey
Insall J N 1984 Surgery of the knee. Churchill Livingstone, Edinburgh
Weightman B 1981 Some engineering principles of joint prosthetics. Br J Hosp Med 25: 285–290

MANAGEMENT OF MAJOR TRAUMA

Immediate management
1. At the site of the accident
    a. Establish and maintain an adequate airway
    b. Control external bleeding by local pressure
    c. Splint fractured limbs using inflatable splints
    d. Consider spinal injury: apply cervical collar or use spinal stretcher
2. In the Accident and Emergency Department
    a. Maintain an adequate airway
    b. Several intra-venous lines are inserted for resuscitation, including a central venous line to measure CVP; typical requirements for blood volume replacement are as follows:
       (i) fractured tibial shaft: 1 unit
       (ii) fractured femoral shaft: 2–4 units
       (iii) major pelvic fracture: 4–6 units
    c. Careful clinical examination
       (i) skull and cervical spine
       (ii) level of consciousness and neurological assessment
       (iii) chest
       (iv) abdomen
       (v) pelvis
       (vi) thoraco-lumbar spine
       (vii) upper and lower limbs

    d. Radiological assessment: the following should be assessed
       in all unconscious victims of road traffic accidents:
         (i) skull
        (ii) cervical spine
       (iii) chest
       (iv) thoraco-lumbar spine
        (v) pelvis
  Other bones should be X-rayed if a fracture is suspected.
    e. Assessment of intra-thoracic and intra-abdominal injuries.
      Refer to Pages 226–231 and 231–234
    f. Splintage of limb fractures
    g. Compound fractures are covered by sterile dressings and
      systemic antibiotics and tetanus prophylaxis given

Common mistakes in immediate management

1. Failure to detect a skull fracture or injury of the cervical or
   thoraco-lumbar spine in an unconscious trauma victim.
   a. All unconscious patients must have radiographs of the skull,
      cervical spine (down to and including C7) and thoraco-
      lumbar spine
   b. These patients should be treated as suffering from a spinal
      injury until proved otherwise
2. Failure to detect a pneumothorax
   a. Chest radiographs may be taken with the patient in a supine
      position and small pneumothoraces secondary to rib
      fractures may be missed
   b. A tension pneumothorax is diagnosed clinically and
      demands urgent attention
3. Failure to adequately replace lost blood volume
   a. There is normally a tendency to under-transfuse most
      trauma patients
   b. This is particularly true if major pelvic fractures are present
4. Failure to detect signs of intra-peritoneal haemorrhage
   a. Symptoms are absent and signs in unconscious patients
      may be masked
   b. Further investigations may be required.
      Refer to Pages 226–227

Management of fractured shaft of femur

Fracture of the shaft of a femur is a major injury and the patient
may suffer hypovolaemic shock.

1. Analgesia
2. 2–4 unit blood volume replacement
3. Radiological assessment of the ipsilateral hip joint is always
   required to exclude an associated dislocation
4. A Denham pin is inserted into the proximal tibia and skeletal
   traction applied
5. Certain fractures especially those of the mid shaft are
   amenable to intramedullary fixation using a Kuntscher nail

Management of pelvic fractures
Fractures involving the ilium or disruption of the pelvic ring result in massive blood loss.
1. Analgesia
2. 4–6 unit blood volume replacement
3. Urogenital damage
   a. Damage to the urethra and bladder may occur following pelvic ring disruption or severe compression fractures
   b. The presence of blood at the external urinary meatus or inability to pass urine should raise the suspicion of urethral damage
   c. Refer to Pages 107–108
4. Paralytic ileus
   a. Common complication of pelvic fractures
   b. Occurs as result of retro-peritoneal haematoma formation
   c. Intra-venous fluids and naso-gastric aspiration are required
5. Sciatic nerve palsy may also complicate severe pelvic fractures
6. Unstable fractures of the pelvic ring
   a. These are best treated by application of an external fixator to relieve pain and facilitate nursing care
   b. Application of a pelvic sling is an alternative
7. Stable fractures of the pelvic ring
   a. Examples include those of the pubic ramus
   b. They are treated as pain allows, non-weight bearing or partial weight bearing on the affected side

Management of spinal injuries and fractures
The possibility of spinal injury should be considered in all unconscious trauma victims. Refer to Pages 218–220

Management of head injuries
1. Detailed assessment of all head injury victims is vital.
2. A full history should be obtained from any witnesses and the ambulance attendants.
3. Examination should pay particular attention to the following points:
   a. Scalp abrasions and lacerations
   b. Depressed skull fractures
   c. Scalp haematomas which may mask or mimick depressed skull fractures
   d. Cerebro-spinal fluid leakage from the nose or ears
4. A full neurological assessment is performed in all patients
5. A history of loss of consciousness following a head injury requires a mandatory overnight admission for observation
6. All unconscious patients must have full radiological examination of the skull and cervical spine

7. Continued head injury observations are essential
   a. Level of consciousness
   b. Pupil size and reaction
   c. Pulse and blood pressure
   d. Respiratory rate
8. Antibiotics are given if a compound fracture is evident or leakage of CSF is present
9. Signs of raised intra-cranial pressure require emergency CT scan
10. Certain depressed skull fractures require elevation and a neurosurgical opinion should be sought

OSTEOMYELITIS

Aetiology
1. Haematogenous infection from a primary focus elsewhere in the body is the commonest cause of acute osteomyelitis in neonates and children
2. In adults the commonest cause is secondary to a compound fracture but infection may also be blood-borne
3. In neonates and children *Staphylococcus aureus* is the commonest organism; streptococci and Gram-negative organisms are seen less commonly
4. In children with sickle cell disease salmonella and *Escherichia coli* infections may be seen
5. In adults a variety of organisms may be found but staphylococci again predominate

Investigations
1. Radiographs of the affected bone may be normal for up to 14 days after the onset of symptoms
2. Full blood count, ESR
3. Chest radiograph
4. Blood cultures
5. MSU
6. Throat swab
7. Isotope bone scan
8. Anti-staphylococcal and anti-streptococcal titres

Treatment
1. Neonatal osteomyelitis
   a. The patient is often septicaemic and requires large doses of parenteral antibiotics such as erythromycin and fusidic acid
   b. If there is no marked improvement within 24 hours surgical exploration and drainage is required to prevent diaphyseal ischaemia

2. Older children and adults
   a. There are proponents for and against early surgery.
   b. Advantages of early surgery include:
      (i) early confirmation of the clinical diagnosis
      (ii) pus is obtained for culture and determination of antibiotic sensitivities
      (iii) early surgical decompression reduces the risk of subsequent ischaemic bone damage
   c. Disadvantages of early surgery are as follows;
      (i) as the patient's general condition is poor it may be preferable to avoid surgery if possible
      (ii) operation is frequently unnecessary for simple subperiosteal infections
      (iii) exploration of the medullary cavity may potentially spread a localised infection
   d. Suggested management:
      (i) Once the diagnosis is suspected the appropriate investigations are performed and parenteral antibiotics are commenced in high doses
      (ii) Erythromycin and fusidic acid are used in combination as first line antibiotic therapy
      (iii) If after 48 hours there are no signs of improvement on clinical assessment, pulse, temperature and ESR, surgical exploration and decompression are performed
      (iv) Antibiotics are altered to suit the sensitivities of the organism isolated
      (v) Antibiotics should be continued for 3 months

Complications
1. Septicaemia which may prove fatal if untreated
2. Acute suppurative arthritis
3. Chronic osteomyelitis which itself has several serious complications:
   a. Chronic discharging sinuses
   b. Sequestrum formation
   c. Bone deformity and pathological fractures
   d. Amyloidosis

Treatment of chronic osteomyelitis
1. Treatment is mainly conservative with antibiotic therapy for acute symptoms
2. Sequestrectomy may be indicated for a persistent discharging sinus
3. A Brodie's abscess is seen radiographically as a cavity with sclerotic margins; treatment is by surgical excision and curettage of the cavity leaving sloping margins in an attempt to prevent further collections of pus

4. Gentamicin beads are now used in chronic bone infection.
   a. Slow release of gentamicin produces high concentrations of antibiotic at the site of infection
   b. A chain of beads is usually removed after 14 days but may be left longer in a cavity

Treatment of osteomyelitis of the vertebral column

1. Infection may be pyogenic caused by *Staphylococcus aureus*, *Escherichia coli*, Klebsiella, Proteus or Pseudomonas sp; Brucella infection should also be excluded in high risk groups
2. The vertebral column is also a common site for tuberculous infection
3. Treatment initially is conservative with bed rest and large doses of parenteral antibiotics even in the presence of neurological impairment
4. A needle biopsy may be useful to identify the causative organism and determine its sensitivities
5. Surgical exploration and decompression is only indicated if there is not a satisfactory response to conservative measures
6. Patients should remain on bed rest for 6 weeks followed by mobilisation wearing a plaster jacket
7. Antibiotics should be continued for 3 months

SEPTIC ARTHRITIS

Aetiology

1. Blood-borne infection from primary focus elsewhere
2. Penetrating injury of joint cavity
3. Secondary to adjacent intra-osseous infection
4. *Staphylococcus aureus* is frequently the causative organism but a variety of other organisms may also be found

Investigations

1. Plain radiographs of adjacent bones
2. Full blood count, ESR
3. Chest radiograph
4. Blood cultures
5. MSU
6. Isotope bone scan
7. Anti-staphylococcal and anti-streptococcal titres

Management

1. Aspirate joint to culture organisms and obtain antibiotic sensitivities
2. If pus is present on aspiration or organisms seen in the aspirate surgical drainage and irrigation of the joint must be performed immediately. There is no place for conservative treatment alone once a diagnosis of septic arthritis has been made

3. Rest affected joint in the position of function
4. High doses of parenteral antibiotics are given.
   a. Erythromycin and fusidic acid are given until the organism and its sensitivities have been identified
   b. Antibiotic therapy should be continued for up to 3 months

FURTHER READING

Silverthorn K G, Gillespie W J 1986 Pyogenic spinal osteomyelitis; a review of 61 cases. NZ Med J 99: 62–65
Thompson D, Bannister P, Murphy P 1988 Vertebral osteomyelitis in the elderly. Br Med J 296: 1309–1311

SPINAL INJURIES

Management of cervical spine injuries
In all unconscious head injury patients a cervical spine injury must be excluded.
1. At site of accident
   a. The head and neck must be carefully supported
   b. A firm cervical collar is applied
   c. An adequate airway must be maintained
   d. No attempt to move the patient is made prior to providing adequate support for the cervical spine
2. In the Accident and Emergency Department
   a. The head and neck are again carefully supported
   b. Radiographs of the cervical spine down to and including C7 are mandatory; if necessary the patient's arms are pulled down to visualise C7
   c. The odontoid peg must also be visualised on the radiographs (The distance between the odontoid peg and the posterior aspect of the arch of the atlas should not be more than 3.0 mm in the adult and 4.5 mm in children)
   d. In the conscious patient flexion and extension views of the cervical spine are obtained. Movements must be performed under medical supervision and stopped immediately if the patient experiences any neurological symptoms in the arms or legs
3. Subsequent management is dependent on whether a fracture is stable or unstable
   a. Stable fractures, e.g. an anterior wedge fracture, are treated with a cervical support collar
   b. Unstable fractures are treated by skull traction
   c. They may need preliminary reduction by traction or less commonly by manipulation especially if facet dislocation has occurred
   d. Traction is applied for a minimum of 6 weeks after which further flexion and extension views are obtained

e. If the fracture remains unstable bone grafting with or without fixation may be required

Management of thoraco-lumbar spine injuries

The possibility of injury to the thoraco-lumbar spine should be considered in all victims of major trauma.

1. At site of accident
   a. All unconscious trauma patients should be treated as a potential spinal injury
   b. Before attempting to move the patient ensure sufficient manpower to support the head and neck, chest, pelvis and limbs
   c. The patient should always be moved 'in one piece' preventing flexion and extension of the spine
   d. The patient is transported on a spinal support stretcher
2. In the Accident and Emergency Department.
   a. Remove all clothing, log rolling the patient 'in one piece'
   b. Examine the spine for abrasions of the overlying skin, haematomas and any palpable step
   c. A complete neurological assessment is performed
   d. Full antero-posterior and lateral radiographs of the thoraco-lumbar spine are mandatory
3. Subsequent management is dependent on whether a fracture is stable or unstable.
   a. Patients with unstable fractures are nursed on a spinal bed such as the circo-electric or Stoke Mandeville bed
   b. The patient is catheterised
   c. Thorough, regular and well recorded assessment of neurological state is essential
   d. Where possible patients should be transferred to a Spinal Injuries Unit
   e. In cases where complete paraplegia is present stabilisation of the fracture using a Hartshill ring or Harrington rods is indicated

Management of traumatic paraplegia

1. Surgical exploration of spinal cord.
   a. Computed tomographic scanning may be used to demonstrate compression of the spinal cord in those patients with partial paraplegia
   b. In these cases surgical exploration, decompression and stabilisation may be indicated
2. Skin care
   a. Pressure sores develop rapidly in anaesthetised skin
   b. Regular turning, washing and drying of the skin are essential
   c. Sheet creases, food crumbs and other foreign bodies should be avoided

3. Bladder function
   a. Intermittent catheterisation under sterile conditions in specialist centres is ideal
   b. Continuous drainage via a silastic urethral catheter is an alternative; catheter blockage must be prevented
   c. Regular urine samples are sent for microscopy and culture
   d. Bladder training is instituted
   e. It may be possible to develop an automatic bladder working reflexly on manual expression
4. Rectal function
   a. Regular enemas are given
   b. Abdominal exercises are encouraged
5. Joints and muscles
   a. Prevention of joint contractures is important
   b. Regular passive movement of all paralysed joints is performed
6. Rehabilitation and restoration of morale
   a. Encouragement and reassurance by all staff is important
   b. Scrupulous attention to hygiene and toilet function is required at all times

BONE TUMOURS

All primary bone tumours are rare. The commonest bone tumour is metastatic spread from a primary malignant tumour at another site. The common primary sites of tumours with secondary spread to bone are:

1. Lung
2. Breast
3. Kidney
4. Prostate
5. Thyroid

Classification of primary bone tumours
1. Tumour-like lesions, e.g. aneurysmal bone cyst, fibrous dysplasia, eosinophilic granuloma
2. Bone-forming tumours, e.g. osteoma, osteoblastoma, osteosarcoma
3. Cartilage-forming tumours, e.g. enchondroma, ecchondroma, chondroblastoma, chondrosarcoma
4. Giant cell tumours
5. Bone marrow tumours, e.g. myeloma, Ewing's tumour
6. Vascular tumours, e.g. haemangioma, angiosarcoma
7. Nervous tissue tumours, e.g. neurofibroma, neurilemmoma
8. Other connective tissue tumours, e.g. lipoma, liposarcoma, fibroma, fibrosarcoma

Investigation of patients with bone tumours
1. Plain radiographs of affected bone
2. Chest radiograph
3. Full blood count, ESR
4. Serum electrophoresis
5. Serum acid phosphatase
6. Bone biopsy
   a. If the diagnosis is in doubt a biopsy is indicated
   b. Incision site of the biopsy must be carefully planned with consideration to any further surgery which may be undertaken once the diagnosis is confirmed
7. Isotope bone scintigraphy
8. Computed tomographic scan of chest
9. Magnetic resonance imaging (MRI) of affected bone which provides a very accurate assessment of the extent of the tumour

Benign bone tumours
1. Tend to occur in adolescents or young adults
2. Radiologically the lesions demonstrate clearly defined margins
3. Benign tumours are usually painfree unless complicated by a pathological fracture
4. Curettage and bone grafting may be required to prevent pathological fracture

Malignant bone tumours
1. Primary malignant bone tumours are often very aggressive
2. Tend to occur in adolescents and young adults
3. Exceptions include osteosarcoma complicating Paget's disease, chondrosarcoma and malignant giant cell tumours
4. Characteristically the patient complains of pain; in patients with vertebral metastases pain at night is typical
5. Radiologically the lesions appear aggressive with ill-defined margins
6. Multimodality treatment is now favoured
   a. Chemotherapy is often given both before and after surgery
   b. In those cases where there is little invasion of adjacent soft tissues amputation is often not required. Limb preservation involves resection of that part of the bone which contains tumour followed by reconstruction using an individually tailored and often extensive endoprosthesis
   c. Adjuvant radiotherapy is important in those patients in whom tumour clearance is minimal

Treatment of osteogenic sarcoma
Osteosarcoma is the commonest of all primary malignant bone tumours. Three quarters arise in the long bones usually of the lower limb and at the site of a metaphysis.

Before the advent of cytotoxic chemotherapy the natural history of osteogenic sarcoma was that 80% of patients would develop pulmonary metastases within a few months of diagnosis. Cade proposed that the primary tumour be treated by radiotherapy and amputation delayed for 6 months and only performed if no pulmonary metastases appeared. The discovery that osteogenic sarcoma is sensitive to high dose methotrexate with folinic acid rescue has changed the treatment fundamentally.

1. After incision biopsy to confirm the clinical diagnosis the patient is treated with three courses of chemotherapy which varies in different centres but always includes high dose methotrexate (HDMTX)
2. After confirming the absence of secondary deposits surgery is then performed. Various possibilities exist:
   a. For tumours in the long bones en bloc wide excision and endoprosthetic replacement is often feasible provided extensive marrow or adjacent soft tissue involvement are not present
   b. If prosthetic replacement is contraindicated limb amputation is required. Amputation must not be performed through the involved bone
   c. Various dispensible bones such as the scapula and ribs can usually be resected without much functional impairment
3. The tumour specimen is carefully examined to determine the percentage of viable tumour cells
4. If the tumour is largely or totally destroyed by the pre-operative chemotherapy the same regimen is continued post-operatively for a further three courses and the patient falls into a favourable prognostic group
5. If the majority of tumour cells appear viable the chemotherapy is changed to a second line regimen and the patient falls into a poor prognostic group

FURTHER READING

Campanacci M, Bacci G, Bertoni F et al 1981 The treatment of osteosarcoma of the extremities; twenty years experience at the Instituto Orthopedico Rizzloi. Cancer 48: 1569–1581
Gitellis S, Bertoni F, Chieti P P et al 1981 Chondrosarcoma of bone. J Bone Joint Surg 63: 1248–1256
Link M P, Goorin A M, Miser A W et al 1986 The effect of adjuvant chemotherapy on disease free survival in patients with osteosarcoma of the extremity. N Engl J Med 134: 1600–1606
Medical Research Council 1986 A trial of chemotherapy in patients with osteosarcoma. Br J Cancer 53: 513–518
Scales J T 1983 Bone and joint replacement for the preservation of limbs. Br J Hosp Med 30: 220–232
Sweetnam D R 1982 Osteosarcoma Br J Hosp Med 28: 112–121
Sweetnam D R 1980 Tumours of bone and their treatment today. Br J Hosp Med 24: 452–465

LOW BACK PAIN

Aetiology

Spinal causes
1. Mechanical causes
   a. Degeneration and displacement (prolapse) of intervertebral disc
   b. Spondylosis
   c. Spondylolisthesis
   d. Scoliosis
   e. Instability syndromes
2. Tumours
   a. Secondary bone tumours especially from primary tumours of the breast, bronchus, prostate, thyroid and kidney
   b. Multiple myeloma
   c. Primary bone tumours
   d. Neural tumours
3. Infection
   a. Discitis
   b. Osteomyelitis, pyogenic or tuberculosis
4. Ankylosing spondylitis
5. Central spinal stenosis
6. Soft tissue ligamentous injuries

Referred back pain
1. Infection of urinary, biliary or female genital tracts
2. Neoplasms of the abdomen or pelvis
3. Abdominal aortic aneurysm

Treatment of prolapsed intervertebral disc

A tear in the annulus fibrosus allows herniation of the nucleus pulposus and is usually secondary to a flexion–rotational injury. The L4/L5 and L5/S1 disc levels are most commonly affected.
  Signs of L5 root compression are:
1. Decreased sensation in L5 dermatome
2. Weakness of extensor hallucis longus
3. Weakness of dorsi-flexion of ankle
4. Wasting of extensor digitorum brevis
  Signs of S1 root compression are:
1. Decreased sensation in S1 dermatome
2. Weakness of plantar-flexion of ankle
3. Weakness of eversion of subtalar joint
4. Absent or diminished ankle jerk
Patients usually present with low back pain, pain in the leg in the L5 or S1 nerve root distribution and tension signs in the leg with limitation of straight leg raising and a positive sciatic stretch test.

1. Conservative treatment
   a. Most patients settle with conservative treatment of which bed rest for 2–3 weeks is most important
   b. Non-steroidal anti-inflammatory drugs (NSAIDs)
   c. Analgesics
   d. Muscle relaxants, e.g. diazepam
   e. Physiotherapy
   f. Epidural analgesia
2. Surgical treatment
   a. Indications for surgery are:
      (i) failure to respond to conservative treatment
      (ii) recurrent acute episodes resulting in loss of work
      (iii) large central disc protrusion causing sphincter disturbance
   b. Prior to surgery radiculography or CT scanning are required to confirm the site of disc protrusion
   c. Operative treatment involves either fenestration discectomy or microdiscectomy
3. Chemonucleolysis
   a. Certain centres use an extract of papain called chymopapain in the treatment of early disc prolapse
   b. This proteolytic enzyme is injected directly into the disc
   c. Anaphylactic reactions have been reported following its use

Treatment of nerve root entrapment syndrome
Entrapment of the nerve roots in the lateral gutters may be due to osteophytic lipping from the posterior facet joints. The presenting features are of sciatic pain in an L5 or S1 nerve root distribution. Straight leg raising is normal with absent tension signs. There is often evidence of chronic nerve root denervation.
1. Conservative treatment
   a. Weight loss
   b. Non-steroidal anti-inflammatory drugs (NSAIDs)
   c. Physiotherapy
   d. Lumbar support corset
2. Surgical treatment
   a. Surgery aims to relieve leg pain in emotionally stable patients who fail to respond to conservative measures
   b. Patients should be investigated by pre-operative nerve conduction studies, radiculography and CT scanning if necessary
   c. Nerve root decompression is performed with undercutting facetectomies

Treatment of central spinal stenosis
Central compression of the cauda equina may be due to hypertrophy of the ligamentum flavum, shingling of the lamina or osteophytic lipping. Patients present with pain in the legs which is

enhanced by walking and associated with muscle weakness. Symptoms tend to abate after resting for 10–15 minutes and especially by sitting. Intermittent claudication due to peripheral vascular disease is an important differential diagnosis. In central spinal stenosis the proximal muscle groups tend to be wasted.

1. Conservative treatment consists primarily of wearing a lumbar support corset
2. Decompressive laminectomy may be required to relieve symptoms

FURTHER READING

MacNab I 1981 Backache. Williams and Wilkins, Baltimore/London

Miscellaneous

ABDOMINAL TRAUMA

Aetiology
1. Road traffic accidents
2. Industrial accidents
3. Civil violence
4. Sporting injuries
5. Iatrogenic injury

Mechanism of injury
1. Penetrating injury
   a. Stab wound
   b. Gunshot or shrapnel wounds due to either low- or high-velocity missiles
2. Non-penetrating injury
   a. Blunt trauma
   b. Deceleration injury
3. Iatrogenic injury

Assessment of intraperitoneal injuries
1. Clinical assessment
   a. Clinical examination of patients following abdominal injury is often difficult
   b. An altered conscious level secondary to a head injury and concurrent chest or skeletal injuries causing hypovolaemic shock may all mask the signs of intra-peritoneal trauma
   c. Measurement of abdominal girth does not provide an accurate measure of the volume of intra-peritoneal blood
2. Investigations
   a. Urinalysis
   b. Erect chest radiograph
   c. Plain abdominal radiographs
   d. Four quadrant abdominal paracentesis
   e. Peritoneal lavage
   f. Serum amylase
   g. Ultrasonography

h. Intravenous urography (IVU)
i. Arteriography
j. Computed tomography

Laparotomy should not be delayed in unstable patients while sophisticated and time-consuming investigations are performed.

Indications for laparotomy

All gunshot wounds of the abdomen should be explored since more than 90% are associated with significant intra-peritoneal injury. While some surgeons advocate exploration of all abdominal stab wounds an increasing number practice selective exploration with a consequent reduction in the negative laparotomy rate. Patients suffering blunt abdominal injuries are managed according to the physical signs present and the results of appropriate investigations. Indications for laparotomy in patients with penetrating and blunt abdominal injuries include:

1. Persistent hypovolaemic shock despite adequate intra-venous fluid replacement
2. Protrusion of a viscus through the abdominal wall
3. Features of generalised peritonitis
4. 'Spleen syndrome' characterised by left shoulder tip pain, left hypochondrial tenderness and fractures of the left lower ribs
5. Free intra-peritoneal gas or fluid on chest or plain abdominal radiographs
6. Free intra-peritoneal blood on four quadrant abdominal paracentesis
7. Positive peritoneal lavage

Surgical management

In those cases where surgery is deemed appropriate a carefully performed and thorough laparotomy is always required as multiple intra-peritoneal injuries are commonly found.

A midline abdominal incision is quick to perform, relatively avascular and can be converted to a thoraco-abdominal incision if required. Penetrating wounds should not be enlarged or extended for exploration; only a formal laparotomy incision allows adequate assessment of all possible intra-peritoneal injuries.

Spleen

The recognition that overwhelming post-splenectomy sepsis (OPSS) is not confined to those undergoing splenectomy as young children but can affect patients splenectomised at any age has stimulated interest in a more conservative approach to splenic trauma. Various techniques of splenorrhaphy have been described.

1. Simple lacerations and capsular tears can often be repaired using absorbable sutures on atraumatic needles
2. Mattress sutures are generally used and can be supported by Teflon buttresses

3. An omental patch may be used to provide additional support for the sutures
4. Topical applications of agents such as gelatin sponge, thrombin, fibrin glue, microfibrillar collagen (Avitene) and mature bovine collagen (Collastat) may prove useful in achieving complete haemostasis
5. In more severe splenic injuries encircling sutures can be passed around the spleen or alternatively it is placed in a prefabricated polyglycolic acid (Dexon) mesh
6. Partial splenectomy with splenic arterial ligation is performed in those cases with damage localised to one area of the spleen
7. Splenectomy is still required in those cases where the spleen is damaged beyond repair or completely avulsed from its pedicle; autologous transplantation of excised splenic tissue into the greater omentum may be performed in these cases

Liver and gall bladder
In general penetrating injuries of the liver have a low mortality as most are caused by stab wounds or low-velocity missiles and result in localised damage of hepatic tissue. In contrast blunt trauma may cause rupture of the liver with severe disruption of the intra-hepatic bile ducts, arteries and veins and devitalisation of large amounts of hepatic tissue. The mortality associated with these injuries is much higher.
1. The objectives of surgical treatment are the arrest of haemorrhage, excision of devitalised liver tissue and provision of adequate drainage
2. Temporary occlusion of the hepatic artery and portal vein by compression of the free edge of the lesser omentum (Pringle's manoeuvre) for a brief period may be used to control torrential haemorrhage from a severely traumatised liver
3. If required hepatic arterial ligation should be accompanied by excision of all devitalised tissue and ligation of the exposed intra-hepatic veins and bile ducts
4. Extensive damage to the liver may require hepatic lobectomy; adequate drainage must always be provided
5. Gauze packing of severe hepatic wounds is used only as a last resort; it allows temporary control of haemorrhage and provides time to transfer a patient to a specialist centre. The pack must always be removed after 24 hours
6. Suturing deep tears of the liver can lead to the intra-hepatic collection of blood, bile and necrotic debris; septic complications frequently follow
7. The common bile duct should not be drained unless it has been injured; routine prophylactic choledochotomy and T-tube drainage in hepatic trauma is of no proven benefit
8. A ruptured gall bladder is usually treated by cholecystectomy

Major blood vessels
Large intra-abdominal blood vessels are rarely injured by blunt trauma but are susceptible to gun shot wounds and stab injuries.
1. Penetrating injuries of the aorta and its main branches are usually fatal and hence seldom seen at operation; they may be sutured primarily or grafted
2. Inferior vena caval injuries are also seldom seen as they too are usually fatal; where possible they should be treated by primary suture but they are notoriously difficult to treat
3. Disruption of the hepatic veins and retro-hepatic vena cava should be suspected when Pringle's manoeuvre fails to control haemorrhage from the liver; unless control of the inferior vena cava can be achieved it is usually a fatal injury
4. Major mesenteric vessels require repair while more peripheral mesenteric vessel injury is managed by resection of the ischaemic bowel

Stomach
1. The lesser sac should always be opened to exclude injury to the posterior wall of the stomach
2. Wounds are closed in two layers using absorbable sutures
3. Post-operative naso-gastric aspiration is required

Pancreas and duodenum
Injuries to the pancreas and duodenum are usually the result of blunt abdominal trauma. A typical example is following high speed impact in a road traffic accident which may crush the duodenum and pancreas between the steering wheel anteriorly and the vertebral column posteriorly. The injury is usually contained within the retroperitoneum and there may be no associated intra-peritoneal injuries. Diagnosis is therefore difficult and often delayed. As a consequence the injury may be difficult to treat.
1. An intra-mural haematoma of the duodenum should be evacuated
2. Small serosal tears of the duodenum should be sutured
3. Where possible full-thickness tears are closed in the transverse axis of the duodenum
4. Larger tears can be closed using a jejunal serosal patch
5. A Roux-en-Y side-to-end duodeno-jejunostomy may be required as an alternative method of duodenal repair
6. Following successful repair of a duodenal injury a feeding jejunostomy may be created or a gastro-jejunostomy fashioned to bypass the injured segment
7. A retro-peritoneal haematoma around the pancreas requires exploration to determine the integrity of the main pancreatic duct

8. A small retro-peritoneal haematoma with superficial contusion or laceration of the pancreas but with the main duct intact is treated by simple evacuation and drainage
9. Major contusion of the distal pancreas with laceration of the pancreatic duct within the body or tail of the pancreas is best treated by distal pancreatectomy and splenectomy; the pancreatic duct is ligated and the proximal remnant oversewn
10. More proximal lacerations of the pancreatic duct can often be treated by subtotal pancreatectomy but pancreatic insufficiency may follow
11. Duodenal diverticulisation is advocated for severe injuries of the pancreatic head; it comprises gastric antrectomy and vagotomy with gastro-jejunostomy and creation of a formal end-duodenal fistula by means of a tube duodenostomy
12. Formation of an internal fistula provides an alternative means of managing such injuries; the proximal end of a Roux loop of jejunum is sutured to the pancreatic head around the site of injury using non-absorbable sutures
13. Pancreatico-duodenectomy (Whipple's operation) may occasionally be required in cases of very severe damage to the pancreatic head and adjacent duodenum

Small intestine
A very detailed examination of the entire small intestine is required. In penetrating injuries perforations of the small intestinal wall are often in pairs and may be hidden in the mesenteric border.
1. Localised perforations or lacerations may be closed primarily
2. More extensive injuries will require small intestinal resection; primary end-to-end anastomosis is usually possible
3. Injury to the small bowel mesentery may lead to devascularisation of a segment of jejunum or ileum necessitating its resection
4. Colon and rectum
   a. The exact nature of the surgical procedure performed will depend on the site and extent of the injury, the degree of peritoneal soiling and the amount of faecal loading within the large bowel
   b. Small wounds of the caecum or colon are exteriorised
   c. More extensive injuries should be treated by resection of the affected segment; conditions are rarely satisfactory for primary anastomosis
   d. Injuries of the rectum and lower sigmoid colon cannot be exteriorised; primary repair is accompanied by a proximal defunctioning colostomy
5. Urinary tract
   Refer to Pages 103–108

FURTHER READING

Bewes P 1983 Open and closed abdominal injuries. Br J Hosp Med
    29: 402–410
Campbell R 1981 Management of pancreatic injuries. Hosp Update 7: 25–33
Cooper M J, Williamson R C N 1984 Splenectomy: indications, hazards and
    alternatives. Br J Surg 71: 173–180
Demetriades D, Rabinowitz B 1984 Selective conservative management of
    penetrating abdominal wounds: a prospective study. Br J Surg 71: 92–94
Henarejos A, Cohen D M, Moossa A R 1983 Management of pancreatic
    trauma. Ann R Coll Surg Eng 65: 297–300
Jones T K, Walsh J W, Maull K I 1983 Diagnostic imaging in blunt trauma of
    the abdomen. Surg Gynecol Obstet 157: 389–398
Oakes D D, Charters A C 1981 Changing concepts in the management of
    splenic trauma. Surg Gynecol Obstet 153: 181–185
Parks T G 1986 Assessment and management of the injured abdomen.
    Postgrad Med J 62: 155–158
Pimpl W, Rieger R, Waclawiczek H W, Thalhamer J 1987 Is the surgical
    preservation of the injured spleen of any use. Surg Res Comm 1: 41–47
Smith J E M 1982 Injuries of the abdomen (1). Hosp Update 8: 145–158
Smith J E M 1982 Injuries of the abdomen (2). Hosp Update 8: 279–286

THORACIC TRAUMA

Aetiology
1. Road traffic accidents
2. Industrial accidents
3. Civil violence
4. Sporting injuries
5. Iatrogenic injuries

Mechanism of injury
1. Penetrating injury
   a. Stab wound
   b. Gun shot or shrapnel wounds
2. Blunt injury
   a. Direct blunt trauma
   b. Deceleration injury
   c. Blast injury
3. Iatrogenic injury

Investigations
1. Erect chest radiograph
   PA, lateral and oblique views
2. Arterial blood gas analysis
   PaO_2, $PaCO_2$ and pH
3. Electrocardiogram
4. Arteriography
5. Computed tomography

Surgical management
1. Fractured ribs
   a. An erect chest radiograph is essential in all cases to exclude an associated pneumothorax or haemothorax
   b. Pain relief is provided by systemic analgesics or intercostal nerve block with a long-acting local anaesthetic, e.g. bupivicaine (Marcain)
   c. Active physiotherapy is required to prevent pulmonary hypoventilation, sputum retention and atelectasis
   d. In severe cases tracheostomy may be required to aid tracheo-bronchial toilet
   e. Fractures of several adjacent ribs may produce a flail segment with paradoxical movement; prolonged intermittent positive pressure ventilation until the segment is stabilised is often needed although primary internal fixation is now an acceptable alternative method of treatment
2. Pneumothorax and haemothorax
   a. May occur after blunt or penetrating injuries
   b. Intercostal underwater seal drainage allows expansion of the collapsed lung and drainage of blood from the pleural cavity
   c. Tension pneumothorax is an important clinical diagnosis requiring immediate intercostal drainage
   d. Indications for thoracotomy include continued haemorrhage, an uncontrolled air-leak indicating a broncho-pleural fistula and a clotted haemothorax
3. Pulmonary contusion
   a. Usually caused by blunt trauma
   b. Localised areas of interstitial haemorrhage and oedema lead to pulmonary atelectasis and impaired respiratory function
   c. Excessive intra-venous fluids may accentuate the degree of pulmonary oedema
   d. Supportive physiotherapy and additional oxygen via a face mask are usually required
   e. Intermittent positive pressure ventilation (IPPV) is needed in cases with severe hypoxia
   f. High dose cortico-steroids, 500 mg methylprednisolone 6-hourly may be of benefit in reducing pulmonary contusion
4. Trachea and bronchi
   a. Tracheal and bronchial injuries are usually the result of blunt trauma
   b. Cough with haemoptysis should suggest the diagnosis
   c. Chest radiographs show mediastinal emphysema if the injury is proximal to the pleural reflection and a pneumothorax in more distal bronchial injuries
   d. Diagnosis is confirmed by bronchoscopy

e. Complete tears of the tracheo-bronchial tree should be repaired surgically; small lacerations can often be managed conservatively

5. Cardiac injuries
   a. Blunt trauma
      (i) Myocardial contusion may produce clinical features, enzyme changes and ECG features typical of an acute myocardial infarction
      (ii) Management is along similar lines
      (iii) More severe blunt trauma may be complicated by contusion, laceration or thrombosis of the coronary arteries or rupture of the ventricular wall, septum or chordae tendinae of the mitral and tricuspid valves; emergency surgical exploration is required in these cases
      (iv) Ventricular aneurysm may present at a later date and also require surgical repair
   b. Penetrating injuries
      (i) Cardiac tamponade is characterised by hypotension, raised venous pressure and quiet or absent heart sounds (Beck's Triad)
      (ii) An initial chest radiograph may be normal but pericardial aspiration reveals blood
      (iii) An emergency thoracotomy is performed through the left fifth intercostal space
      (iv) The pericardium is incised anterior to the phrenic nerve
      (v) Blood and blood clot are evacuated from the pericardial sac and the cardiac laceration sutured using non-absorbable sutures
      (vi) The sutures must be placed carefully so as not to occlude the coronary vessels

6. Thoracic aorta
   a. An acute deceleration injury may cause a partial tear of the aortic arch just beyond the origin of the left subclavian artery; below this point the descending thoracic aorta is relatively fixed
   b. A haematoma may be temporarily contained by the aortic aventitia or periaortic tissues; this false aneurysm may occasionally organise to form a traumatic aneurysm but more often the haematoma ruptures usually within 7–10 days
   c. The femoral pulses may be weakened or delayed and a recurrent laryngeal nerve palsy may be evident
   d. Chest radiographs show widening of the superior mediastinum and possibly a left haemothorax
   e. The diagnosis is confirmed by aortography or CT scanning
   f. Repair is undertaken through a left thoracotomy using a prosthetic graft

7. Diaphragm
   a. Lacerations of the diaphragm caused by penetrating injuries should be sutured using non-absorbable material
   b. Rupture of the diaphragm producing a traumatic diaphragmatic hernia usually occurs on the left side allowing the stomach and other viscera to pass into the pleural cavity and producing a characteristic radiographic appearance
   c. Typically the diaphragmatic tear is radial extending from the oesophageal hiatus
   d. Passage of a naso-gastric tube will allow a distended, herniated stomach to deflate thus minimising the respiratory embarrassment
   e. Repair of a ruptured diaphragm may be undertaken via either the abdominal or thoracic approach; laparotomy allows a more detailed and complete examination of the abdominal viscera
   f. Accurate apposition of the torn margins of the diaphragm is achieved using non-absorbable sutures

Prognostic factors in thoracic trauma
The following features are associated with increased morbidity and mortality following chest injury.
   1. Extreme of age
   2. Pre-existing pulmonary or cardiac disease
   3. Previous chest surgery
   4. Obesity
   5. Deformity of chest wall or thoracic spine

FURTHER READING

Demetriades D, Rabinowitz B, Markides N 1986 Indications for thoracotomy in stab injuries of the chest: a prospective study of 543 patients. Br J Surg 73: 888–890
Fleming H A 1983 Nonpenetrating trauma and the heart. Hosp Update 9: 995–1006
Moussalli H, Hooper T 1986 Management of chest injuries: 1. Hosp Update 12: 751–760
Moussalli H, Hooper T 1986 Management of chest injuries: 2. Hosp Update 12: 880–896

PROPHYLAXIS OF POST-OPERATIVE SURGICAL WOUND INFECTION

Infection of a surgical wound is associated with increased post-operative morbidity and increases a patient's duration of hospital stay. More serious post-operative infections such as intra-peritoneal abscess formation and septicaemia are associated with an increased post-operative mortality. In addition wound infection predisposes to other complications including stitch sinus formation, dehiscence and incisional herniation. Appropriate measures must always be taken to minimise post-operative sepsis.

Factors predisposing to wound infection
1. Host resistance
   a. General factors
      (i) age
      (ii) obesity
      (iii) uraemia
      (iv) jaundice
      (v) malnutrition
      (vi) diabetes
      (vii) hypovolaemic shock
      (viii) hypoxia
      (ix) anaemia
      (x) malignant disease
      (xi) corticosteroid, cytotoxic and anti-metabolite drugs
   b. Local factors
      (i) impaired vascularity
      (ii) haematoma and seroma formation
      (iii) necrotic tissue
      (iv) foreign bodies
      (v) previous irradiation
2. Microbial contamination
   a. type and virulence of organism
   b. size of bacterial inoculum
   c. pattern of resistance to antibiotics and antiseptics

Incidence of postoperative wound infection
Wound sepsis following surgery may be the result of either endogenous or exogenous bacterial contamination of the operative wound. The majority of wound infections following abdominal surgery are caused by endogenous contamination and the wound infection rate is directly related to the degree of per-operative contamination.

Type of surgical wound	Wound infection rate (%)
Clean	<2
Clean/contaminated	10
Contaminated	15
Infected	40

Prevention of exogenous wound infection
1. Correct autoclaving of surgical instruments, drapes and theatre gowns

2. Adequate skin cleansing prior to putting on sterile gowns and gloves and adherence to strict aseptic techniques
3. Positive pressure ventilation of operating theatres with use of high efficiency particulate air filters
4. Laminar clean air flow chambers, e.g. Charnley tent
5. Identification and treatment of operating theatre personnel carrying *Staphylococcus aureus*

Prevention of endogenous wound infection
1. Skin preparation
   a. Shaving, clipping or depilating skin
   b. Antiseptics, e.g. iodine, chlorhexidene gluconate
   c. Adhesive drapes, e.g. Opsite
2. Mechanical bowel preparation
   a. Low residue diet followed by clear fluids
   b. Oral aperients, e.g. magnesium sulphate, magnesium citrate and sodium picosulphate (Picolax)
   c. Osmotic purgatives, e.g. mannitol, polyethylene glycol
   d. Pre-operative whole gut perfusion with Ringer-lactate or other isosmolar electrolyte solutions
   e. Per-operative (on-table) antegrade colonic irrigation
3. Oral antibiotics
   a. Oral administration of antibiotics that are poorly absorbed by the gastro-intestinal tract has a maximal effect on the faecal flora with minimal risk of systemic toxic effects·
   b. Should not be given for more than 24 hours pre-operatively as resistant bacteria are likely to emerge within the colon and pseudo-membranous colitis may develop
   c. Unsuitable for patients with intestinal obstruction and others requiring emergency surgical procedures
   d. Neomycin–metronidazole and neomycin–erythromycin are popular combinations of oral antibiotics given prior to elective colorectal surgery
4. Intra-incisional antibiotics or antiseptics
   a. Topical application of antibiotics or antiseptics to the edges of the wound immediately prior to its closure may reduce the incidence of wound infection but it will have no effect on other septic complications such as intra-peritoneal abscess formation
   b. Local infiltration of antibiotics into the site of a surgical incision immediately prior to start of an operation achieves a high concentration of antibiotic within the tissues around the surgical wound during the course of the operation; further infiltration is required if the wound is extended
5. Systemic antibiotics
   a. Given by intra-venous injection at the time of induction of anaesthesia to ensure high tissue levels of the antibiotic during the surgical procedure

b. In colorectal surgery systemic antibiotics are generally more effective than oral antibiotics in preventing wound infection
c. If contamination has been severe or the operative procedure prolonged a further dose of antibiotic is given
d. Further prolongation of prophylactic antibiotic therapy does not influence the rate of wound infection and may serve to select resistant organisms
e. The choice of antibiotic should reflect the probable contaminating organisms and their usual sensitivities
f. For gastric and biliary surgery a cephalosporin is usually sufficient
g. For appendicectomy and colorectal surgery a cephalosporin or aminogylcoside should be combined with metronidazole
6. Peritoneal lavage
   a. Saline
   b. Povidone–iodine
   c. Tetracycline solution (1 mg/ml saline)
7. Surgical technique
   a. Avoid spillage of gastro-intestinal contents
   b. Surgical wound isolators
   c. Isolation of infected or contaminating organs – 'danger towel' technique

Special situations
1. Implantation of prosthetic materials
   a. Infection of implanted prosthetic material usually has disastrous consequences
   b. Complete elimination of infection is normally only possible if the infected prosthesis is removed
   c. Although recognised as clean operations with a relatively low wound infection rate replacement arthroplasty and insertion of prosthetic heart valves and synthetic arterial grafts should always be covered by prophylactic antibiotics
   d. All patients should receive an antibiotic with activity against *Staphylococcus aureus* and the common Gram-negative aerobic organisms; a cephalosporin is usually used
2. Amputation of the lower limb
   a. Following lower limb amputation for peripheral vascular disease infection by Clostridial organisms is a major hazard and is potentially fatal
   b. Penicillin and metronidazole are the commonly used prophylactic agents

FURTHER READING

Editorial 1980 Prophylaxis of surgical wound spesis. Br Med J (i): 1063–1064

Hunt T K 1981 Surgical wound infections: an overview. Am J Med
    70: 712–718
Johnson C D, Kelly M J, Mortensen N J McC 1987 Mechanical
    contamination and surgical technique in gastrointestinal anastomoses.
    Surg Res Comm 1: 147–150
Keighley M R B 1983 Perioperative antibiotics. Br Med J 286: 1844–1846
Krukowski Z H, Matheson N A 1983 The management of peritoneal and
    parietal contamination in abdominal surgery. Br J Surg 70: 440–441
Persson U, Montgomery F, Carlsson A, Lindgreen B, Ahnfelt L 1988 How far
    does prophylaxis against infection in total joint replacement offset its
    cost? Br Med J 296: 99–102
Pollock A V 1988 Surgical prophylaxis – the emerging picture. Lancet
    1: 225–229

CRYOSURGERY

Introduction
Freezing of viable tissues to treat various disease states is called
cryosurgery. Tissue destruction by cryosurgery now has many
applications. The rapid freezing of living cells produces various
cytotoxic effects
1. Intra-cellular ice crystal formation leads to puncturing of cell
   membranes
2. Denaturation of cell membrane lipid-protein complexes.
3. Extra-cellular ice crystal formation produces accumulation of
   hyperosmolar electrolyte solutions within the adjacent cells
4. Microvascular stasis and thrombosis leading to cellular
   hypoxia

Techniques
1. Application of liquid nitrogen produces a tissue temperature of
   approximately −180°C and its use is generally confined to the
   treatment of small, superficial skin lesions
2. Closed nitrous oxide cryoprobes produce tissue temperatures
   of approximately − 80°C and are suitable for most benign and
   pre-malignant lesions
3. Large vascular lesions often require use of a liquid nitrogen
   probe to produce sufficient cryonecrosis
4. The temperature of the cryoprobe is monitored using a
   thermocouple
5. Freezing for 1 minute is usually sufficient for benign lesions on
   mucosal membranes; 2 minutes are normally required for
   lesions on squamous surfaces
6. Most cryoprobes now have a heating coil to allow rewarming
   following cryodestruction
7. The configuration of the cryolesion is determined by the size
   and shape of the cryoprobe
8. The depth of the lesion is determined by compression of the
   cryoprobe against the lesion or its elevation once adhesion has
   been achieved

9. When treating vascular lesions occlusion of feeding vessels by digital compression facilitates cryosurgery
10. Preliminary infiltration with a vasoconstrictor such as adrenaline solution also reduces vascularity and shortens the duration of freezing required

Indications
Cryosurgery is often the treatment of choice for benign and pre-malignant lesions situated on accessible mucosal surfaces. It may also be useful in the palliation of recurrent malignant disease at these sites but it does not usually have a role in the treatment of primary invasive carcinoma.

1. Benign conditions
   a. Vascular lesions, e.g. telangiectases, haemangiomata
   b. Various benign lesions of the buccal mucosa, e.g. compound papillomas, fibroepithelial polyps, mucous retention cysts and fibrous epulides
   c. Warts, perianal and penile condylomata
   d. Pyogenic (infective) granuloma
   e. Second and third degree haemorrhoids
   f. Chronic cervicitis and cervical erosions
   g. Urethral caruncle
   h. Tonsillectomy in patients with coagulation disorders such as haemophilia and von Willebrand's disease
   i. Trans-cranial or trans-sphenoidal hypophysectomy
   j. Lens extraction in cataract surgery
2. Pre-malignant lesions
   a. Leukoplakia
   b. Bowen's disease
   c. Rectal polyps
3. Malignant lesions
   a. Basal cell carcinomas (rodent ulcers) especially where multiple lesions are present (Gorlin's syndrome)
   b. Control of recurrent cervical carcinoma of the vault of the vagina
   c. Palliative treatment of residual or recurrent carcinoma of the oral cavity effectively controls pain, infection and haemorrhage
   d. Palliative treatment of rectal carcinoma
   e. Primary treatment of invasive tumours such carcinoma of the uterine cervix or oral cavity in very elderly, frail or severely debilitated patients where conventional treatment is thought to be unsuitable

Advantages of cryosurgery
1. Treatment is simple and can usually be performed as an outpatient
2. Anaesthetic is often not required

3. Biopsy can be taken at the time of cryosurgery
4. Minimal post-operative discomfort occurs as there is little surrounding tissue response and nerve endings are destroyed
5. Post-operative oedema, infection and haemorrhage are rare
6. Scarring is minimal and the cosmetic result is usually as good if not better than conventional surgical treatment or radiotherapy
7. Cryodestruction of malignant tissue may possibly initiate a specific immune response

LASER SURGERY

Introduction
1. A laser (Light Amplification by Stimulated Emission of Radiation) is a unique form of coherent monochromatic light of intense energy which liberates heat on contact with a suitable surface and can be used to cut, coagulate or vapourise tissue
2. The effects of laser energy depend on three features
   a. Wavelength: determined by the source of the laser
   b. Power density: dependent on the power of the laser source, the size of the beam and the distance between the source and the target
   c. Absorption and scatter: related to the type of tissue, its colour and the presence of specific pigments, e.g. melanin, haemoglobin

Characteristics of individual lasers
Three types of laser are used clinically:

	Wavelength (μm)	Power (W)	Tissue penetration (mm)
Argon	0.5	1–20	0.5
Carbon dioxide	10.6	1–300	0.2
Neodymium-YAG	1.1	1–100	2.0

Advantages
1. High-energy beam can be focussed to a small spot size; this allows precision with little surrounding tissue damage
2. Direct contact with tissues not required
3. Lasers can be delivered via flexible fibres and therefore can be used endoscopically

Applications
1. Ophthalmology
   a. Diabetic retinopathy
   b. Retinal tears

2. Otolaryngology
   a. Carcinoma and polyps of larynx
   b. Laryngeal stenosis
   c. Stapedectomy in otosclerosis
3. Neurosurgery
   a. Excision of intra-cranial tumours
   b. Destruction of intra-cerebral tumours
4. Dermatology
   a. Treatment of haemangiomas and telangiectasia
   b. Removal of papillomas, tattoos, warts and cutaneous
      secondary deposits
5. Gastroenterology
   a. Palliative treatment of obstructing oesophageal carcinomas
   b. Control of haemorrhage from peptic ulcers and inoperable
      gastric carcinomas
   c. Haemostatic scalpel in liver resection
6. Gynaecology
   a. Vapourisation of abnormal epithelium or cone biopsy for
      carcinoma in situ
   b. Division of adhesions in Fallopian tube surgery
   c. Destruction of endometriosis at laparoscopy
7. Thoracic surgery
   a. Tracheal and bronchial strictures
   b. Palliative treatment of obstructing bronchial tumours

Hazards
1. Potential dangers to the patient's and operator's eyes require
   elaborate precautions including wearing safety glasses and use
   of non-reflective instruments
2. Accidental fires caused by ignition of PVC tubing and
   inflammable anaesthetics which must not be used with lasers
3. Ignition of rectal gas
4. Perforation of hollow viscus

FURTHER READING

Cochrane J P S 1986 Lasers in surgical practice. In: Russell R C G (ed)
   Recent advances in Surgery, Vol 12. Churchill Livingstone, Edinburgh
   pp 17–27
Nussbaum M, Ghazi A 1986 Endoscopic applications of laser surgery. In:
   Nyhus L M (ed) Surgery Annual. Appleton-Century-Crofts, Norwalk,
   Connecticut pp 225–241
Swain C P, Bown S G, Edwards D A W, Kirkham J S, Salmon P R, Clark C G
   1984 Laser recanalisation of obstructing foregut cancer. Br J Surg
   71: 112–115
Vallon A G 1982 Lasers and fibreoptic endoscopy. Br J Hosp Med
   27: 175–179

METABOLIC RESPONSE TO SURGERY AND TRAUMA

Any injury to the body is associated with a complex metabolic response mediated by various neural and hormonal reflexes. The response is regulated by centres within the hypothalamus and is effected mainly via the sympathetic nervous system. The principle individual metabolic responses to injury and their hormonal mediation are shown below.

Catabolic phase

1. Water and electrolyte metabolism (increased aldosterone and anti-diuretic hormone (ADH))
   a. Increased urinary potassium excretion
   b. Decreased urinary sodium excretion
   c. Decreased urinary water excretion
2. Protein metabolism (increased catecholamines)
   a. Increased breakdown of skeletal muscle protein
   b. Reduced protein anabolism
   c. Increased urinary nitrogen excretion
3. Fat metabolism (increased catecholamines)
   a. Increased lipolysis
   b. Increased levels of circulating free fatty acids
4. Carbohydrate metabolism (increased levels of glucagon, cortisol, thyroxine, growth hormone and catecholamines)
   a. Increased glycogenolysis and gluconeogenesis
   b. Increased blood sugar levels with impaired glucose tolerance due to insulin antagonism
   c. Increased basal metabolic rate
5. The catabolic or 'flow phase' of the metabolic response to injury is accompanied by increased energy expenditure and a negative nitrogen balance which lead to a loss of body weight
6. The size and duration of the response are directly related to the severity of the trauma or magnitude of the surgical procedure
7. The most dramatic changes are seen after severe trauma with multiple fractures and extensive burns
8. If sepsis complicates surgery or trauma a further increase in the metabolic response is seen

	Daily urinary excretion			Duration of response (days)
	Basal state	Moderate trauma	Severe trauma	
Water (litres)	1.5	1.0	0.5	1–2
Sodium (mmol)	70	5–10	1	2–5
Potassium (mmol)	70	100	140.	1–3
Nitrogen (g)	10	15–20	20–30	4–10

Anabolic phase
1. At the end of the catabolic phase these changes are reversed and an anabolic or 'recovery phase' commences
2. This lasts until the body has fully recovered from the initial injury

The metabolic response to injury is a physiological response but persistence of the catabolic phase causes delayed wound healing and increased susceptibility to infection which reduce the chances of survival.

FURTHER READING

Elwyn D H, Kinney J M, Askanazi J 1981 Energy expenditure in surgical patients. Surg Clin N Am 61: 545–556

PARENTERAL NUTRITION

Parenteral nutrition is essential to the survival of many surgical patients but it is an expensive form of therapy costing at least £50–70 per patient per day. In addition it is not without its own complications and therefore should not be used unless specific indications exist. Most patients require intra-venous nutrition for only a limited period of time. A few will require prolonged or indefinite therapy which can often be administered at home.

Indications
1. Gastro-intestinal failure (patients who can't eat)
   Parenteral nutrition may be used before surgery as well as in the post-operative period, e.g.
   a. oesophageal obstruction
   b. gastric outlet obstruction
   c. prolonged paralytic ileus
   d. inflammatory bowel disease
   e. radiation enteritis
   f. short bowel syndrome
   g. gastro-intestinal fistulae
   h. acute pancreatitis
2. Hypermetabolic states (patients who can't eat enough)
   Parenteral nutrition is often used to supplement enteral feeding in patients with severe catabolic states, e.g.
   a. severe burns
   b. septicaemia and other serious infections
   c. major trauma
3. Anorectic states (patients who won't eat)
   Patients with anorexia due to malignant disease, especially during chemotherapy or radiotherapy, may occasionally require parenteral nutritional support

Nutritional requirements

Total parenteral nutrition (TPN) aims to provide all the body's daily
requirements via the intra-venous route.

1. Energy
   Various substrates of different calorific values are used to
   provide energy, e.g.

Substrate	Calorific value (kcal/g)
Carbohydrate	4
Fat	9
Protein	4

   Energy requirements are determined by the degree of the
   body's catabolism (kcal/kg body weight/day)

Basal state	Moderate catabolism	Severe catabolism
30	35–40	40–60

2. Nitrogen
   The nitrogen requirements of an intra-venous feeding
   regimen are supplied by various amino acids. As with energy
   requirements those of nitrogen are related to the severity of the
   patient's catabolic state: (mg/kg body weight/day)

Basal state	Moderate catabolism	Severe catabolism
160	200–300	300–500

3. Water: 2500–3000 ml/day
4. Electrolytes
   a. Sodium (80–100 mmol/day)
   b. Potassium (60 mmol/day)
   c. Calcium (10–20 mmol/day)
   d. Magnesium (15–30 mmol/day)
   e. Chloride (100 mmol/day)
   f. Phosphate (15–50 mmol/day)
5. Vitamins
   a. Water-soluble vitamins
      Vitamin B_1 (thiamin) (3.0 mg/day)
      Vitamin B_2 (riboflavin) (3.6 mg/day)
      Vitamin B_6 (pyridoxine) (4.0 mg/day)
      Vitamin B_{12} (cobalamin) (5 μg/day)
      Niacin (40 mg/day)
      Pantothenic acid (15 mg/day)
      Biotin (60 μg/day)
      Folic acid (0.4 μg/day)
      Vitamin C (ascorbic acid) (100 mg/day)

   b. Fat-soluble vitamins
     Vitamin A (1000 μg/day)
     Vitamin D (5 μg/day)
     Vitamin E (10 mg/day)
     Vitamin K (70 μg/day)
6. Minerals (Trace elements)
   Iron (20–70 μmol/day)
   Copper (5–25 μmol/day)
   Zinc (40–90 μmol/day)
   Manganese (5–15 μmol/day)
   Selenium (0.4 μmol/day)
   Molybdenum (0.2 μmol/day)
   Iodine (1–7 μmol/day)
7. Essential fatty acids

Parenteral nutritional regimens

1. Carbohydrate
   a. Glucose (dextrose), the physiological carbohydrate, is the most commonly used carbohydrate energy source: impaired utilisation may require additional insulin therapy
   b. Fructose is converted by the liver into glucose prior to utilisation and must only be given to patients with normal hepatic function: lactic acidosis and hypophosphataemia are important complications
   c. Maltose has a low renal threshold and large amounts may be lost in the urine producing an osmotic diuresis
   d. Alcohols such as ethanol and sorbitol, the alcohols of glucose and fructose respectively, are both liable to produce lactic acidosis and are therefore no longer used routinely: their use is contraindicated in liver and renal disease

2. Fat
   a. Intralipid (500 ml of 20% solution or 1000 ml of 10% solution daily) is an aqueous emulsion of soya bean oil which contains glycerol, phosphate and phospholipid plus essential fatty acids including linoleic, linolenic, oleic, palmitic and stearic acids and vitamin E
   b. A daily limit of 30 ml/kg body weight of 10% solution or 15 ml/kg body weight of 20% solution should not be exceeded
   c. Utilisation may be impaired in critically ill patients; failure to clear the infused lipid leads to persistent lipaemia
   d. Intralipid should be avoided in patients with severe liver disease and those with haemorrhagic diatheses

3. Nitrogen
   a. Amino acid solutions were originally derived from protein hydrolysates but various mixtures of synthetic crystalline amino acids are now available

    b. Their exact composition varies but all contain the essential amino acids and most mimic the amino acid content of proteins with a high biological value

    c. Examples of commercially available amino acid solutions include Aminofusin, Aminoplex, Synthamin and Vamin

    d. Each solution can be supplied with various concentrations of the constituent amino acids, e.g. Synthamin 9, 14, 17, the suffixing numbers indicating the different nitrogen concentrations (g/l)

4. Minerals (trace elements)
   Addamel (10 ml daily) provides calcium (5 mmol), magnesium (1.5 mmol), iron (50 μmol), zinc (20 μmol), manganese (40 μmol) and copper (5 μmol) plus fluoride (50 μmol), iodide (1 μmol) and chloride (13.3 μmol) ions

5. Vitamins
   a. Solvito (1 vial daily) provides the water soluble vitamins B and C plus nicotinamide, biotin and folic acid
   b. Vitlipid (10 ml daily) provides the fat soluble vitamins A, D and K

Routes of administration

1. Central venous feeding
   a. Hyperosmolar solutions must be administered directly into a central vein where they are rapidly diluted by the fast flow of blood to avoid thrombosis and thrombophlebitis
   b. Insertion of a central venous catheter by percutaneous puncture of the subclavian vein via an infraclavicular approach is the most popular route of administration
   c. The tip of the catheter should lie in the superior vena cava
   d. For long-term parenteral nutrition a Hickman or Broviac catheter is inserted into the subclavian vein via the cephalic vein in the delto-pectoral groove

2. Peripheral venous feeding
   a. Lower osmolality solutions may be administered via peripheral veins
   b. Infusion thrombophlebitis limits the duration of peripheral venous feeding at each site to 3–4 days

Catheter related complications

1. Air embolism
2. Pneumothorax
3. Sepsis
4. Subclavian arterial injury
5. Brachial plexus injury
6. Thoracic duct laceration
7. Intra-pleural infusion of nutrient solution
8. Pericardial tamponade
9. Catheter embolism

10. Venous thrombophlebitis, thrombosis and pulmonary embolism

Metabolic complications
1. Hyperglycaemia (diabetes mellitus)
2. Hyperglycaemic nonketotic hyperosmolar coma
3. Rebound hypoglycaemia
4. Lactic acidosis
5. Essential fatty acid deficiency
6. Hypokalaemia
7. Hypophosphataemia
8. Hyperammonaemia
9. Vitamin, mineral and trace element deficiencies
10. 'Fat overload' syndrome

Precautions
1. Strict aseptic technique essential when inserting central venous catheter
2. Patient positioned with a 20–30° head-down tilt when inserting catheter
3. Silicone catheter tunnelled subcutaneously on anterior chest wall to reduce incidence of catheter sepsis
4. Confirm position of catheter tip with PA chest radiograph prior to infusion of nutrient fluids
5. Protect catheter entry site with local antiseptic cream and occlusive dressing
6. Catheter dressing and intra-venous giving set changed at regular intervals with full aseptic technique
7. Luer hub locking avoids accidental disconnection of intra-venous giving set from catheter
8. Central venous catheter should not be used for administering drugs, blood transfusion, withdrawing blood samples or measuring central venous pressure
9. Three-litre bags which contain the fluid and nutritional requirements of each 24 hour period are prepared under aseptic conditions using a laminar air flow screen
10. An electronic volumetric pump is used to accurately regulate the infusion of nutrient solutions
11. Pulse and temperature should be recorded at 4-hourly intervals while parenteral nutrition is being administered
12. Remove central line if catheter infection is suspected; take blood cultures through the catheter and culture its tip on removal
13. Strict adherence to clinical and laboratory monitoring of patient by a multi-disciplinary nutritional care team

Monitoring

Careful monitoring is required to prevent the complications associated with parenteral nutrition and to ensure an adequate response to the feeding regimen.

1. Clinical monitoring

Parameter	Frequency
Temperature and pulse	4-hourly
Urinalysis	6-hourly
Fluid balance	daily
Body weight	weekly

2. Laboratory monitoring

Parameter	Frequency
Haemoglobin	daily
White cell count	daily
Prothrombin time	weekly
Urea/creatinine	daily
Serum electrolytes	daily
Blood glucose	daily
Calcium and phosphate	daily
Urinary nitrogen	daily
Serum albumin	weekly
Liver function tests	weekly

As the patient's condition improves and his nutritional requirements become stabilised the frequency at which these parameters are measured can be reduced.

FURTHER READING

Pettit S H 1985 Clinical nutrition: intravenous feeding. Hosp Update 11: 533–545
Editorial 1986 Central venous catheterisation. Lancet ii: 669–670
Goodgame J T 1980 A critical assessment of the indications for total parenteral nutrition. Surg Gynecol Obstet 151: 433–441
Haddock G, Barr J, Burns H J G, Garden O J 1985 Reduction of central venous catheter complications. Br J Parenteral Therapy 6: 124–128
Hatfield A R W 1982 Hyperalimentation. Br J Hosp Med 28: 220–233
Jackson M A 1983 Long-term home parenteral nutrition. Br J Hosp Med 29: 105–116
Johnston I D A 1979 Hazards of intravenous feeding. Adverse Drug Reaction Bull 77: 276–279
Lennard-Jones J E, Wood S 1985 The organisation of intravenous feeding at home. Health Trends 17: 73–75
MacFie J 1986 Towards cheaper intravenous nutrition. Br Med J 292: 107–108

MacFie J 1984 Active metabolic expenditure of gastroenterological surgical patients receiving intravenous nutrition. JPEN 8: 371–376
Mughal M, Irving M 1986 Home parenteral nutrition in the United Kingdom and Ireland. Lancet ii: 383–386

LAPAROSCOPY

Laparoscopy is commonly used by most gynaecologists for both diagnostic and therapeutic procedures. The technique is also applicable to several surgical conditions.

Indications
1. Liver disease
2. Abdominal mass
3. Ascites
4. Investigation of acute abdominal pain
5. Pre-operative staging of gastric and lower oesophageal carcinomas

Contra-indications
1. Haemorrhagic diathesis
2. Previous abdominal surgery other than appendicectomy through a right iliac fossa incision
3. Tense ascites
4. Generalised peritonitis
5. Sepsis of the anterior abdominal wall
6. Gross obesity
7. Cardio-respiratory failure

Technique
1. Usually performed under general anaesthesia with endotracheal intubation and muscle relaxation
2. Local anaesthetic infiltration can be used in selected patients
3. The bladder must be drained prior to laparoscopy
4. Pneumoperitoneum is established by insufflation of the peritoneal cavity with 2–3 litres of carbon dioxide through a Verres needle
5. The laparoscope is inserted via a sub-umbilical stab incision
6. A palpating probe is inserted through a separate stab incision to manipulate the mobile intra-peritoneal structures and permit full examination of the peritoneal cavity and its contents
7. Target biopsy of the liver may be performed using a Menghini needle; diagnostic accuracy is greater than blind percutaneous biopsy using a 'Tru-cut' needle
8. Other intra-peritoneal lesions can be biopsied using grasping forceps and small scissors
9. A cholangiogram can be obtained by inserting a fine needle through the abdominal wall and the right lobe of the liver to puncture the hepatic surface of the gall bladder

Complications
Laparoscopy is usually a relatively safe procedure. Complications occur in 1–5% of examinations but the mortality rate should be less than 0.1%.
1. Subcutaneous emphysema
2. Mediastinal emphysema
3. Air embolism
4. Haemorrhage
5. Perforation of small or large intestine, bladder, etc.

Advantages of laparoscopy over laparotomy
1. Lower morbidity and mortality than laparotomy
2. Unnecessary laparotomy is usually avoided
3. Cheaper investigation than laparotomy requiring a much shorter period of hospitalisation

FURTHER READING

Clarke P J, Hands L J, Gough M H, Kettlewell M G W 1986 The use of laparoscopy in the management of right iliac fossa pain. Ann R Coll Surg Eng 68: 68–69
Deutsch A A, Zelikorsky A, Reiss R 1982 Laparoscopy in the prevention of unnecessary appendicectomies: a prospective study. Br J Surg 69: 336–337

TUMOUR MARKERS

Characteristics
1. A tumour marker is any substance that is related to the presence or progress of a tumour
2. Not all markers are tumour-specific
3. Tumour markers may be secreted by tumours into the blood or serous fluids (serum tumour markers) or expressed on the surface of tumour cells (tissue tumour markers)
4. Tumour-derived markers are actually produced by a tumour, either the malignant cells or stromal cells. They may represent excessive secretion of a normal cellular product (e.g. calcitonin in medullary carcinoma of the thyroid gland) or the production of a substance not normally produced by the tissue concerned (e.g. adreno-corticotrophic hormone by oat cell tumours of the lung)
5. Tumour-associated markers are produced by non-malignant cells as a result of the presence of a tumour (e.g. increased urinary hydroxyproline excretion in skeletal metastases)
6. Tumour markers are assayed by various methods often involving radio-immunoassay

7. Tumour markers may be of value in the following clinical situations:
   a. Diagnosis
   b. Screening
   c. Estimation of tumour bulk and staging
   d. Tumour localisation
   e. Assessment of prognosis
   f. Prediction of response to treatment
   g. Measurement of response to treatment
   h. Detection of recurrence after treatment
8. Tumour markers commonly used in clinical oncology are tabulated below

Serum tumour markers

Marker	Tumour	Value
Beta human chorionic gonadotrophin (β-HCG)	Chorio-carcinoma	a, b, c, e, f, g, h
	Testicular teratoma	a, b, c, e, g, h
Alpha feto protein (AFP)	Hepatoma	a, g, h
	Testicular teratoma	a, b, c, e, g, h
Carcino-embryonic antigen (CEA)	Colo-rectal carcinoma	c, d, e, g, h
Paraproteins	Myelomatosis	a, c, g, h
Acid phosphatase	Prostatic carcinoma	a, c, e, g, h

Eutopic hormones
(Normal hormones produced in excessive quantities from normal site of origin)

Parathormone (PTH)	Parathyroid adenoma	a, d
ACTH	Cushing's disease	a, d
GH	Pituitary adenoma	a
Calcitonin	Medullary thyroid carcinoma	a, b, g, h
Insulin	Insulinoma	a, b, d, g, h
Catecholamines	Phaeochromocytoma	a, b, d
Gastrin	Gastrinoma	a, b, c, d, g, h
5-HT	Carcinoid tumour	a, d, g, h
Erythropoietin	Hypernephroma	g, h

Ectopic hormones
(Normal hormones produced in excess from abnormal sites)

ACTH	Bronchial	e, f
ADH	and	
PTH	breast	
Calcitonin	carcinomas	

Tissue tumour markers

Marker	Tumour	Value
Oestrogen receptors (ER)	Breast carcinoma	e, f,
Epithelial membrane antigen (EMA)	Epithelial carcinomas	a
Carcino-embryonic antigen (CEA)	Breast carcinoma Bronchial carcinoma	a
T-cell/B-cell markers	Lymphomas Leukaemias	a a, e
Common-ALL antigen	Acute lymphoblastic leukaemia	e, f
HLe-1	Reticulo-endothelial tumours	a

FURTHER READING

Bagshawe K D 1984 Clinical applications of hCG. Adv Exp Med Biol 176: 313–324

Begent R H J 1987 The value of carcinoembryonic antigen in clinical practice. Br J Hosp Med 37: 335–338

Buckman R 1982 Tumour markers in clinical practice. Br J Hosp Med 27: 9–20

Horwich A 1984 Serum tumour marker regression rate following chemotherapy for malignant teratoma. Eur J Cancer Clin Oncol 20: 1463–1470

Light P A 1985 Tumour markers in testicular cancer. J R Soc Med 78 Suppl 6: 19–24

Rustin G J 1986 Tumour markers in germ cell tumours. Br Med J 292: 713–714

SKIN GRAFTS, FLAPS, AND FREE TISSUE TRANSFERS

Skin grafts, skin flaps and free tissue transfers are used to reconstruct cutaneous defects which cannot be closed primarily. Composite flaps have a role in reconstructing other soft tissue defects and bones.

Skin grafts

All skin grafts need to obtain an adequate blood supply from the recipient site and therefore cannot be applied to tendon, bare bone or cartilage

1. Split-thickness (Thiersch) skin grafts
   a. An easily performed one-stage technique but the skin graft may be rapidly destroyed by infection especially Group A β-haemolytic streptococci
   b. Contraction may impair the subsequent cosmetic appearance thus preventing their use on the face
   c. A meshed skin graft increases the area which it can be used to cover
2. Full-thickness (Wolfe) skin grafts
   a. Skin must be cleared of all subcutaneous fat to ensure the graft's success
   b. A one-stage procedure is possible and a good cosmetic result can be obtained but only small areas of skin can be grafted
   c. Donor sites commonly used are the post-auricular region and the supra-clavicular fossa

Skin flaps

A skin flap retains its subcutaneous fat with an integral blood supply.

Random pattern skin flaps

These have a random blood supply and as a result length:width ratios greater than 1:1 are associated with distal necrosis.

1. Local transposition flaps
   a. Examples include rotation and advancement flaps
   b. A one-stage procedure is possible using skin of the same or similar quality to that from which the defect arose
   c. Sensation is usually preserved
2. Cross-transfer flaps
   a. Examples include cross-finger or cross-leg flaps
   b. They also allow reconstruction with similar skin
   c. Immobilisation of both the donor and recipient digit or limb is required and consequently these flaps have declined in popularity
3. Tube pedicle flaps
   a. Formed by two adjacent flaps of 1:1 ratio and sewn up as a tube
   b. By a series of delayed transfers the tube can be moved to any site
   c. Prolonged immobilisation in awkward positions may be required
   d. Multiple operations are required over several months to achieve the end result

e. Haematoma formation may impair the vascularity of the graft and cause distal ischaemia with shortening of the tube

f. Now rarely used in reconstructive surgery

Axial pattern flaps
1. Skin flap is supplied by a named artery and vein which form a vascular pedicle and allow a large area of skin to be used
2. Length:width ratio can exceed 1:1
   a. Delto-pectoral (Bakamjian) flap is based on the perforating branches of the internal thoracic (mammary) artery and vein
   b. Forehead flap is supplied by the anterior division of the superficial temporal artery
3. Provided the flap is handled carefully it usually survives well

Free vascular flap
1. An area of skin with its arterial blood supply and accompanying venous drainage is mobilised, detached and transferred to the recipient site
2. The flap is revascularised by microvascular anastomoses to suitable vessels at the recipient site
3. Groin flap
   a. Provides skin based on the superficial circumflex iliac artery and vein
   b. Despite obtaining a relatively large area of skin the donor site can often be closed directly leaving a relatively inconspicuous scar
4. Dorsalis pedis free flap
   a. Skin of the dorsum of the foot is supplied by the dorsalis pedis artery and drained by the short and long saphenous veins
   b. The donor site is covered by a split-thickness skin graft
   c. Flap is useful for reconstructing facial defects after excision of skin for burns

Free vascular flaps provide a single-stage procedure which allows transfer of large areas of full-thickness skin to any site on the body surface. Microvascular anastomoses demand special skills and expertise in addition to expensive equipment. Prolonged operating times are usually required. Flap failure is normally due to arterial or venous thrombosis. In the absence of complications hospitalisation is greatly reduced when compared with multi-stage skin transfer techniques such as tube-pedicle transfer.

Composite flaps
Composite flaps comprise skin plus underlying structures such as muscle and bone and have an integral blood supply. They may be used as local transpositional or free vascularised flaps.

1. Myocutaneous flaps
   a. Small perforating vessels pass from the muscle to the overlying skin and ensure its viability
   b. Latissimus dorsi myocutaneous flap consists of the skin of the postero-lateral chest wall plus underlying latissimus dorsi muscle: it is supplied by the thoraco-dorsal artery which arises from the subscapular artery, and is used to reconstruct large defects of the neck and chest wall and in breast reconstruction following mastectomy. Primary closure of the skin defect is usually achieved
   c. Rectus abdominis myocutaneous flap can be based on either the inferior epigastric vessels to reconstruct thigh, groin or perineal defects or the superior epigastric vessels to reconstruct chest wall defects and for breast reconstruction
   d. Pectoralis major myocutaneous flap is supplied by the pectoral branch of the thoraco-acromial artery and is used in head and neck reconstruction including reconstruction of the oro-pharynx
2. Osseo-cutaneous flaps
   a. The iliac crest or deep circumflex iliac flap comprises a portion of the iliac crest along with the overlying skin: it is supplied by the deep circumflex iliac artery and vein and is used in the treatment of ununited tibial fractures and mandibular reconstructions
   b. Radial forearm flap is based on the radial artery and its accompanying veins and contains a segment of distal radius; it is useful in reconstructing defects of the mandible and it supplies skin which is similar in texture to that of the oral mucosa

FURTHER READING

Asko-Seljavaara S, Lahteenmaki T, Waris T, Sundell B 1987 Comparison of latissimus dorsi and rectus abdominis free flaps. Br J Plast Surg 40: 620–628

Bailey B N 1979 Latissimus dorsi flaps – a practical approach. Ann Acad Med 8: 445–453

Breach N M 1986 Oropharyngeal reconstruction. 1. Cutaneous and myocutaneous flap repair. In: Bloom H J G, Hanham I W F, Shaw H J (eds) Head and Neck Oncology. Raven Press, New York pp 109–111

Goldwyn R M 1987 Breast reconstruction after mastectomy. New Eng J Med 317: 1711–1714

Harrison D H 1980 Microvascular surgery: free flap transfer. Hosp Update 6: 235–245

Hayden R E 1986 Role of microvascular surgery in head and neck reconstruction. In: Bloom H J G, Hanham I W F, Shaw H J (eds) Head and Neck Oncology. Raven Press, New York pp 65–72

Jones B M 1985 Predicting the fate of free tissue transfers. Ann R Coll Surg Eng 67: 63–70

Webster M H C, Soutar D S 1986 Practical Guide to Free Tissue Transfer. Butterworths, London

MICROSURGERY

Introduction

Microsurgical techniques continue to be developed in many surgical specialities. The feature common to all microsurgery is the use of very fine instruments and sutures (6/0–10/0) which necessitate the use of an operating microscope or magnifying loupes.

1. Ophthalmology
   a. Keratoplasty
   b. Cataract extraction
   c. Prosthetic lens implantation
   d. Trabeculectomy drainage for glaucoma
   e. Vitrectomy
2. Otolaryngology
   a. Stapedectomy
   b. Fenestration
   c. Tympanoplasty
   d. Microlaryngoscopy
3. Neurosurgery
   a. Ligation of intra-cranial aneurysms
   b. Excision of spinal cord tumours
   c. Excision of acoustic neuromas
4. Urology
   a. Reversal of vasectomy
   b. Orchidopexy for high undescended testis
5. Gynaecology
   a. Reversal of tubal ligation or diathermy
   b. Colposcopy
6. Microvascular surgery
   a. Replantation of limbs or digits following traumatic amputation
   b. Digital auto-transplantation
   c. Free transfer of vascularised skin flaps, muscles or bone either individually or as composite grafts in reconstructive surgical procedures. Refer to Pages 254–255
   d. Auto-transplantation of small intestine for pharyngo-oesophageal replacement
   e. Extracranial–intracranial revascularisation: Refer to Page 148
7. Microneural surgery
   a. Primary and secondary nerve repair by inter-fascicular suture
   b. Anastomosis of nerves to produce useful sensory and motor function in auto-transplanted digits and replanted digits and limbs

Advantages
1. The magnified view of the operating field allows tissues to be examined more easily: using a binocular microscope stereoscopic vision is preserved
2. Microsurgery enables dissection, mobilisation and suturing to be performed with great accuracy: trauma to the structures within the operating field is therefore minimised
3. Assistants and observers have the same view of the operating field as the surgeon which facilitates teaching
4. Television camera can be used to record operative procedures

Disadvantages
1. Equipment, especially the operating microscope, is quite expensive
2. Considerable experience is required to attain and maintain an adequate level of expertise
3. Great care must always be taken and this is often reflected in the long duration of microsurgical operations

FURTHER READING

Birchall J P, Hattab M, Pearman K, Mathias D B, Black M J M 1983 Microvascular free jejunal transfer reconstruction following pharyngo-laryngectomy. Ann R Coll Surg Eng 65: 209–211

Davies D M 1985 Microvascular surgery. Br Med J 290: 910–912

Emerson J 1981 Peripheral nerve injury. Hosp Update 7: 595–605

Harrison D H 1980 Microvascular surgery: replantation. Hosp Update 6: 381–389

Harrison D H, O'Neill T J 1980 Microvascular surgery: basic techniques. Hosp Update 6: 149–161

Kester R C, Leveson S H 1981 A Practice of Vascular Surgery. Pitman, London pp 191–209

Rich W J 1977 Microsurgery. In Taylor S (ed) Recent Advances in Surgery Vol 9. Churchill Livingstone, Edinburgh pp 191–208

MONOCLONAL ANTIBODIES

Monoclonal antibodies can be produced to a wide variety of antigens, especially tumour-associated antigens, using the mouse hybridoma technique. This method produces large quantities of monoclonal antibody of high specificity from a single cell line in tissue culture which can be maintained indefinitely.

Production
1. Hybridoma cells are produced by fusion in polyethylene glycol of malignant myeloma cells with antibody-producing splenic B-lymphocytes from mice immunised with a specific antigen

2. Hybrid cells are cultured for two weeks and the secreted monoclonal antibodies extracted from the supernatant culture medium
3. Hybridoma cells are cloned on soft agar to produce single cell lines
4. Selected hybridoma cells are maintained in cell culture to produce monoclonal antibodies or by injection into the peritoneal cavity of syngeneic mice

Advantages
1. The antigen binding site of each monoclonal antibody is homogenous and highly specific to the antibody binding site of the particular antigen
2. No contamination by non-specific antibodies
3. Immunisation of mice with impure antigenic material allows production of antibodies to previously unknown antigens
4. A limitless supply of each specific monoclonal antibody permits their widespread use and detailed standardisation

Diagnostic uses
1. Immuno-histopathological diagnosis
   a. Differentiation between various tumours such as malignant lymphoma and anaplastic carcinoma is often not possible using routine histological stains
   b. Monoclonal antibodies can be used to identify the antigenic markers of several tumours by immuno-histochemical techniques
   c. Differentiation between lymphomas, malignant melanoma, breast carcinoma and tumours of the gastro-intestinal tract is now possible as each exhibits specific cell surface antigens for which monoclonal antibodies have been prepared
2. Serological diagnosis
   a. Levels of circulating tumour-associated antigens such as alpha-feto protein, carcino-embryonic antigen and chorionic gonadotrophin are usually measured using conventional polyclonal antisera
   b. Radio-immuno assays utilising monoclonal antibodies are now used in preference as they have greater specificity
   c. Monoclonal antibodies have also been used to identify and characterise various additional antigens such as Ca 19–9 and Ca 125 in the serum of patients with malignant disease
3. Tumour localization
   a. Gamma camera imaging allows localization of tumours which take up specific monoclonal antibodies labelled with radionuclides
   b. Although both primary and secondary tumours can be shown by this technique it is likely to be most useful in the detection and localization of recurrent disease

   c. The technique is possible with conventional antisera but monoclonal antibodies have far fewer cross reactions and hence greater specificity

   d. Reduced antigen expression by certain tumours will produce false negative results

Therapeutic uses

Several possibilities exist for the use of monoclonal antibodies in treating patients with malignant disease.

1. In vitro use in patients with systemic disease requiring high-dose chemotherapy or radiotherapy:
   a. Elimination of contaminating malignant cells from bone marrow suspensions prior to autologous bone marrow transplantation
   b. Elimination of T-lymphocytes from bone marrow suspensions prior to allogeneic bone marrow transplantation in an attempt to prevent graft-versus-host disease (GVHD)
2. In vivo use is likely to cause sensitisation and allergic reactions as monoclonal antibodies are foreign proteins.
   a. Unmodified monoclonal antibodies may exert a cytostatic or cytotoxic effect on malignant cells exhibiting a specific tumour antigen
   b. Monoclonal antibodies can be modified by coupling with high energy radionuclides, chemotherapeutic agents or cellular toxins to increase their therapeutic potential; by delivering the coupled agent directly to the tumour its systemic toxicity should be reduced

FURTHER READING

Allum W H, MacDonald F, Fielding J W L 1986 Monoclonal antibodies in the diagnosis and treatment of malignant conditions. In: Nyhus L M (ed) Surgery Annual. Appleton-Century-Crofts, Norwalk, Connecticut pp 41–64

Armitage N C 1986 The localization of anti-tumour monoclonal antibodies in colorectal cancer. Ann R Coll Surg Eng 68: 302–306

Armitage N C, Perkins A C, Durrant L G et al 1986 In vitro binding and in vivo localization in colorectal cancer of a high affinity monoclonal to carcinoembryonic antigen. Br J Surg 73: 965–969

Beverley P C L 1983 Monoclonal antibodies. Hosp Update 9: 223–228

Hardcastle J D, Baldwin R W 1986 Monoclonal antibodies. In: Russell R C G (ed) Recent Advances in Surgery Vol 12. Churchill Livingstone, Edinburgh pp 43–64

Makin C A 1986 Monoclonal antibodies raised to colorectal carcinoma antigens. Ann R Coll Surg Eng 68: 298–301

Rainsbury R M 1984 The localisation of human breast carcinomas by radiolabelled monoclonal antibodies. Br J Surg 71: 805–812

Williams M R, Perkins A C, Campbell F C et al 1984 The use of monoclonal antibody 791T/36 in the immunoscintigraphy of primary and metastatic carcinoma of the breast. Clin Oncol 10: 375–381

BURNS

Aetiology

1. Thermal
   a. Wet – contact with hot liquid or gas (scald)
   b. Dry – flash or flame contact (burn)
2. Electrical
   a. Full-thickness burns occur at the sites of entry and exit of the electrical current
   b. High voltage current may cause extensive tissue necrosis between the entry and exit sites
3. Chemical
   a. Chemical burns may continue to progress in depth and severity even when the causative agent has apparently been removed
   b. Phenol (carbolic acid) and its derivatives are particularly dangerous
   c. Many chemicals produce systemic toxicity such as metabolic alkalosis or acidosis and renal or hepatic damage
4. Ionising radiation
   a. Radiation burns are often more extensive than initially suspected
   b. The systemic effects of excessive radiation such as bone marrow depression are often delayed

Depth of burn

1. Partial-thickness burns
   a. Superficial burns
      (i) Loss of the epidermis and the superficial layers of the dermis
      (ii) Area heals spontaneously usually within 14 days and with minimal scarring
   b. Deep dermal burns
      (i) Only the deepest epithelial components such as the sweat glands and hair follicles are preserved
      (ii) Vascular supply is precarious and the burn may easily be converted into a full-thickness burn if it becomes infected or oedematous
      (iii) Spontaneous healing does occur but it is slow and results in hypertrophic scarring and is often complicated by significant contractures
2. Full-thickness (deep) burns
   a. No dermal epithelium is retained
   b. Skin grafting is always required and in the case of exposed bone, tendon or joint capsule a skin flap is necessary

The immediate appearances of a wound are often deceptive depending on the nature of the mechanism of the burn. Usually a burn that is red and moist is superficial. A white dry area indicates a deep dermal burn. Full-thickness burns are usually leathery in appearance. Pin prick sensation is lost in full-thickness burns but this test is not always reliable. Thermography reveals areas where the cutaneous plexus of vessels is destroyed or where blood flow is arrested due to intra-vascular coagulation. This too is not always accurate.

Area of burn

1. Determination of the area of the burn allows calculation of the intra-venous fluid requirements
2. The 'Rule of Nines' is frequently used but it is inaccurate in children especially in those less than 1 year old as the head and neck have a proportionately larger surface area than in adults
3. The Lund and Browder chart provides a more accurate assessment of the area of the burn
4. The palmar surface of the patient's hand represents approximately 1% of the body surface area

Prognosis

1. Mortality increases with age and is also related to the patient's previous state of health especially the presence of chronic cardio-respiratory disease
2. As a rough guide if the patient's age in years plus the percentage area of burn exceeds 100 the chances of survival are very poor
3. Pulmonary injury secondary to inhalation of smoke, hot gases and steam is also associated with a marked reduction in survival

Immediate management of the burned patient

1. Extinguish flames, remove heat source or burning agent and isolate from electrical source
2. Ensure adequate airway and oxygenation
   a. Humidified oxygen via face mask is given to all patients who have inhaled hot gases or smoke
   b. Endotracheal intubation may be required in cases of laryngeal oedema; tracheostomy is best avoided unless oral endotracheal intubation is not possible
   c. Intermittent positive pressure ventilation (IPPV) with positive end-expiratory pressure (PEEP) is required for those with pulmonary oedema
   d. Blood gas analysis is required to monitor oxygen therapy and ventilatory requirements
3. Cool burnt area
   a. Put burnt area in cold bath or under running water
   b. Copious lavage is required if chemicals are present on the skin surface
4. Apply clean dressing to burnt area

5. Intra-venous fluid replacement therapy
   All adults with greater than 15% burns and children with greater than 10% burns must be admitted to hospital and will require intra-venous fluids
   a. Crystalloid solutions
   b. High molecular weight dextrans (Dextran 110) in saline
   c. Modified gelatin plasma expanders (Gelofusine, Haemaccel)
   d. Plasma protein fraction (PPF)
   e. Plasma
   Various formulae have been devised to calculate the intra-venous fluid requirements. In addition to the calculated requirements 2 litres of glucose water must be given for the patient's metabolic requirements. Where possible this is given orally; if not the intra-venous route is used.
   Muir and Barclay Formula:
      Ration of human plasma is calculated from the formula:
   Ration (ml) = surface area of burn (%) × body weight (kg) × 0.5
      Plasma is given intra-venously over 36 hours following the burn:
   a. 3 rations are given in the first 12 hours
   b. 2 rations are given in the following 12 hours
   c. 1 ration is given in the final 12 hours
   Evans (Roehampton) Formula:
      120 ml of Dextran 110 is given for each 1% surface area burned over 48 hours in the following aliquots:
   a. 50% in first 8 hours
   b. 25% in next 16 hours
   c. 25% in final 24 hours
   Brooke Formula:
   a. During first 24 hours: 1.5 ml Ringer lactate plus 0.5 ml colloid per kg body weight for each 1% surface area burned
   b. During second 24 hours: half the above amount adjusted according to urine output

6. Monitor fluid replacement therapy
   The various formulae available provide a rough guide to the rate at which intra-venous fluids should be infused. Careful monitoring of the following parameters allows maintenance of an adequate plasma volume for correct tissue perfusion:
   a. Pulse, blood pressure and central venous pressure
   b. Hourly haematocrit (packed cell volume) from which the circulating plasma deficit or excess can be calculated
   c. Urine output must exceed 0.5 ml/kg body weight per hour and ideally should exceed 1.0 ml/kg body weight per hour

7. Analgesia
   a. Self administration of Entonox (50% nitrous oxide; 50% oxygen may be useful initially)
   b. Small doses of narcotic analgesics such as morphine 5 mg or pethidine 50 mg should be given intra-venously

   c. Further doses are usually required at frequent intervals; a
      continuous infusion of opiate analgesics may be more
      satisfactory
   d. Analgesics given by intra-muscular injection have an
      unpredictable effect and should not be given by this route
 8. Escharotomy
   a. Circumferential burns of the chest may inhibit ventilation
      while those of the limbs may cause peripheral ischaemia
      and even gangrene
   b. Early longitudinal division of constricting eschars avoids
      these complications
 9. Tetanus prophylaxis is given to patients not adequately
    immunised
10. Blood transfusion
   a. Whole blood is not given within the first 24 hours of injury
      as haematocrit estimations could no longer be used to
      accurately monitor fluid replacement therapy
   b. Blood transfusion is rarely required for patients with partial-
      thickness burns
   c. In patients with full-thickness burns which exceed 10% of
      the body's surface area 1% of the patient's normal blood
      volume is transfused for each 1% area of full-thickness burn
11. Systemic antibiotics
   a. Routine use of prophylactic systemic antibiotics does not
      reduce the incidence of sepsis and should be avoided
   b. If used they are liable to promote the growth of resistant
      bacteria and lead to colonisation by various yeasts and
      fungal organisms

Later management of the burned patient
Having provided adequate resuscitation within the first 48 hours
following injury the care of the patient is aimed at maintaining a
good nutritional status despite the presence of a highly catabolic
state.
 1. Patient is nursed in a warm environment (24–26°C) to minimise
    surface energy losses by evaporation, especially if the patient's
    burns are being treated by exposure
 2. High calorie and protein intake
   a. Fine-bore naso-gastric tube feeding may be used to
      supplement an increased oral diet; mineral and vitamin
      supplements are often given
   b. Parenteral nutrition may be required in patients with severe
      hypercatabolic states who are unable to take or absorb
      sufficient nutrients via the enteral route
 3. Blood transfusion may be required to correct anaemia
 4. Once the patient has been discharged from hospital an
    appropriate programme of rehabilitation is followed

Local management of the burn

The aims of local care of the burned area are to prevent further tissue loss and to aid rapid healing whilst minimising infection, scarring and secondary deformity.

1. Exposure techniques
   a. Must be performed in the controlled environment of a purpose built burns unit
   b. With exposure to the air the burn exudate forms a dry crust which prevents infection
   c. The exposed surface must be kept dry and cracks prevented
   d. Useful for facial, perineal burns and any situation where it is difficult to apply dressings
   e. Various techniques are available:
      (i) open bed with sterile linen changed at frequent intervals
      (ii) sterilised polyurethane foam
      (iii) support from a net bed
      (iv) levitation on an air-loss bed
   f. Laminar air flow is an important factor in preventing infection
   g. If the burnt areas have not crusted and dried by about 48 hours dressings are required to prevent infection
2. Conventional dressing techniques
   a. Dressings should be applied and changed under strict aseptic conditions
   b. Vaseline impregnated gauze is covered by several layers of absorptive dressings
   c. Adhesive polyurethane film (Op-site) is useful for small areas of superficial skin loss
   d. Antibacterial creams can be applied directly to the burn surface and covered by absorptive dressings
      (i) 1% silver sulphadiazine (Flamazine) cream
      (ii) Mafenide acetate (Sulfamylon) cream
   e. 0.5% silver nitrate soaked dressings, which must be kept moist by repeated applications of the silver nitrate solution, provide good prophylaxis against infection by Pseudomonas species
3. Early surgical excision and skin grafting
   a. Deep dermal or full thickness burns are excised with a skin grafting knife until healthy tissue is reached (tangential excision)
   b. Excision is usually performed between the 2nd and 5th days after the burn occurred
   c. Area of excision is then grafted usually with an unexpanded split thickness skin graft
   d. Temporary cover prior to definitive skin grafting may be provided by allografts (fresh or deep frozen human skin) or xenografts (sterilised, lyophilised pig skin)

4. Delayed skin grafting
   a. Performed after about 14 days when the eschar is separating and the final thickness of the burn has been definitely established
   b. Following excision of the eschar a meshed split thickness skin graft is usually applied
5. Pressure garments to reduce hypertrophic scarring
6. Physiotherapy and occupational therapy to aid return of function
7. Delayed reconstructive surgery
   a. Surgical correction of unpleasant scars and contractures may require a series of operative procedures
   b. It is often delayed for up to 18 months after the original injury

FURTHER READING

Brown J, Ward D J 1984 Immediate management of burns in casualty. Br J Hosp Med 31: 360–368

Harvey Kemble J V 1980 Management of burn wound and sepsis. Hosp Update 6: 1057–1064

Settle J A D 1982 Fluid therapy in burns. J R Soc Med 75 Suppl 1: 6–11

Sutherland A B 1985 Nutrition and general factors influencing infection in burns. J Hosp Inf 6 Suppl B: 31–42

ACQUIRED IMMUNE DEFICIENCY SYNDROME (AIDS)

Introduction
1. Caused by a T cell lymphotrophic retrovirus identified as HTLV-III or HIV (Human Immunodeficiency Virus) which infects specific target cells
2. AIDS virus possesses a reverse transcriptase enzyme which enables its genetic structure to become permanently incorporated into the nuclei of infected cells; division of infected cells produces more active virus particles
3. Virus is detected by a specific antibody test
4. A characteristic reversal of the T-helper to T-suppressor (T4/T8) cell ratio is seen in AIDS

High-risk groups
1. Homosexual and bisexual men
2. Intra-venous drug abusers
3. Haemophiliacs
4. Haitians and Central Africans

Clinical features
1. Kaposi's sarcoma and other malignant neoplasms
2. Opportunistic infections

Infecting organisms causing opportunistic infection
1. Fungal
   a. *Candida albicans*; mouth, oesophagus, lung
   b. *Cryptococcus neoformans*; lung, central nervous system
   c. Histoplasma; lung
   d. Aspergillus; lung, central nervous system
2. Protozoal
   a. *Pneumocystis carinii*; lung
   b. *Toxoplasma gondii*; lymph nodes, brain
   c. Cryptosporidia; gastro-intestinal and biliary tracts
3. Bacterial
   a. Mycobacterium avium-intracellulare; lung, lymph nodes, gastro-intestinal tract, central nervous system
   b. Mycobacterium tuberculosis; lung
   c. Salmonella; gastro-intestinal tract, septicaemia
4. Viral
   a. Cytomegalovirus (CMV); central nervous system, gastro-intestinal tract
   b. Herpes simplex; gastro-intestinal tract, central nervous system

Indications for surgery in patients suffering from AIDS
Surgical intervention is usually required to obtain either tissue or fluid for culture or tissue for histological examination.
1. Bronchoscopy
   a. Broncho-alveolar washings
   b. Trans-bronchial lung biopsy
2. Lymph node biopsy
3. Brain biopsy
4. Laparotomy
5. Long-term venous access for antimicrobial therapy and parenteral nutrition

Precautions
1. Assume all patients in high risk categories are infected with HIV.
   a. Incubation period and length of time for seroconversion are unknown and may be quite long
   b. Screening all patients in high risk groups is not feasible
2. Basic precautions should be those taken when operating on patients known to carry hepatitis B virus
3. Pass sharp instruments and needles using a dish or tray rather than from hand to hand
4. Needle stick injuries should be washed well and encouraged to bleed
5. If accidental injury occurs an immediate blood sample is taken to confirm negative HIV antibody status followed by a further sample at 3 months to determine whether or not seroconversion has occurred

FURTHER READING

Cohen J 1984 AIDS – a review. Br J Hosp Med 31: 250–259

Curran J W 1985 The epidemiology and prevention of the acquired immune deficiency syndrome. Ann Intern Med 103: 657–662

Melbye M 1986 The natural history of human T lymphotrophic virus-III infection: the cause of AIDS. Br Med J 292: 5–12

Pinching A J 1988 Clinical aspects of AIDS and HIV infection in the developed world. Br Med Bull 44: 89–100

Pinching A J, Weiss R A, Miller D 1988 AIDS and HIV infection: new perspective. Br Med Bull 44: 1–19

Tedder R S 1988 HIV testing: problems and perceptions. Br Med Bull 44: 161–169

Sim A J W, Dudley H A F 1988 Surgeons and HIV. Br Med J 296: 80

Index